MW00648536

VITAMIN D DEFICIENCY

AND COVID-19

Its central role in the word pandemic

VITAMIN D DEFICIENCY AND COVID-19

Its central role in the word pandemic

Drs David C Anderson and David S Grimes

© Drs David C Anderson and David S Grimes, 2020

Published by Tennison Publishing

All rights reserved. No part of this book may be reproduced, adapted, stored in a retrieval system or transmitted by any means, electronic, mechanical, photocopying, or otherwise without the prior written permission of the author.

The rights of Drs David C Anderson and David S Grimes to be identified as the authors of this work have been asserted in accordance with the Copyright, Designs and Patents Act 1988.

A CIP catalogue record for this book is available from the British Library.

ISBN 978-0-9562132-7-3 (Paperback)
ISBN 978-0-9562132-8-0 (ePub)
ISBN 978-0-9562132-9-7 (Mobi)

Book layout and cover design by Clare Brayshaw

Prepared and printed by:

York Publishing Services Ltd
64 Hallfield Road
Layerthorpe
York YO31 7ZQ

Tel: 01904 431213

Website: www.yps-publishing.co.uk

Contents

Introduction

2020 will be remembered as a pivotal year, or perhaps just a catastrophic year in which the pinnacle of prosperity was reached. The growth of the second half of the 20th century was remarkable, a wonderful era to live through, not just for economic, but also for scientific development. Medicine made enormous advances with greater understanding of physiology, how the body works. This included remarkable genetic understanding, with the discovery of the double helix of DNA in 1953. There were technological advances in medicine with the introduction of open heart surgery, kidney dialysis, intensive care units and much else. Neonatal and maternal deaths in Britain fell to almost zero. The humanitarian aspect of medicine also improved, with the development of hospices and specialised care of the elderly.

The early 21st century became the era of the financial whizz-kids with vast bonuses to supplement very big incomes. But excessive de-regulation and greed within the financial services led to a serious economic crisis in 2008. Recovery was almost complete by the start of 2020, but no-one could foresee the enormous economic collapse that was to occur over just the first few months. In the new era of the Personal Computer, Facebook, a Twittering President, massive commercial jets, and infinite communication, sudden collapse seemed to Oldies like us to be at the same time both unthinkable and inevitable.

But whence and how was it going to come? Then in an instant there it was, collapse triggered by the pandemic of Covid-19. Throughout the winter a minute virus had been probing for our species' weakest points and blind spots, and had found them all at once, in the form of a unique mix of human stupidity and widespread deficiency of Vitamin D.

A bit about the authors

We are two retired physicians in apparent good health and in our late seventies, whose paths first crossed over 40 years ago in the Manchester Royal Infirmary. We next bumped into one another in a virtual sense in April 2020 during the coronavirus pandemic, on which we have a very similar Vitamin D-orientated perspective. When we first met fleetingly half a lifetime ago, Manchester Medical School was right at the centre of research into Vitamin D, in the form of Professor Bill Stanbury, and his team of researchers under the unassuming but imaginative direction of the late Dr Barbara Mawer. Barbara died of cancer aged just 70 in March 2006, and were she still alive she would undoubtedly have brought her knowledge and skills, which extended from the lab into Liberal politics, to bear on Covid-19 and its attendant sanctimonious cant. She was interested in all aspects of the Sunshine Vitamin; but in her absence we have to fill in as best we can.

Put in a nutshell we are convinced that the Covid-19 pandemic has been and still is being approached in a way that is fundamentally flawed through ignorance and much wilful neglect of some basic Vitamin D-related biology. Though we humans often behave as though we are gods, we too are an animal species and so all about biology, for whom things will always break down at the weakest link. A particularly weak philosophical point here has been to treat this viral infection as a powerful and vicious external enemy, while ignoring fundamentals.

Viruses are simply partial life forms that use our bodies to replicate and spread their DNA or (as in this case) RNA. And a successful virus does not kill the hand that feeds it (that is you and I); why kill the very being on which you depend? The most successful RNA viruses cause the common cold, whereby the virus and our bodies have evolved an understanding which allows us to survive, while the virus just gets to do its own thing, which is to propagate itself. So here we will try and explain where we each came from, and explore together where we believe our species should be going to get out of the global viral mess.

Unfortunately politicians, and often those in charge of medical politics, belong to a different species, *Homo politicans,* that lives as if above and beyond normal biological considerations. But to mix metaphors, some virological chickens are now coming home to roost. And it may be up to us Oldies, who have forgotten how to remain ignorant of mere facts, to understand and propagate the right lessons from the current pandemic pandemonium, and extract *Homo sapiens* from the quick-sands of Covid-19. We started to write this on 12th May 2020. Time inevitably hangs on our hands during so-called 'lockdown', so we set out to finish it by the end of the month, a mere 20 days away. In the first instance it is only going to be available as an E-book. But the idea is to make it as informative for ourselves as for you, dear reader, and together to try to sketch out a sensible path forward.

We start with the text of a short Youtube film that one of us (DA) made and published on Youtube on March 22nd 2020, the day after the Spring Equinox.

An Endocrinologist's advice: wise up on Vitamin D: *Coronavirus may know more about it than you do.*

Viruses are partial life forms that use our bodies to multiply and spread their personal RNA or DNA. It is tough luck if you die in the process, but don't blame the virus for just doing its own thing. Blame yourself, or, better, learn something about Vitamin D that COVID-19 may already 'know'.

Our distant sun-worshiping forebears took the Spring Equinox very seriously, maybe in part because of an essential chemical called Vitamin D3, or cholecalciferol. Only the Sun's UV rays can act on our skin to break the B ring of dehydrocholesterol and so form Vitamin D. The liver then makes the storage form, 25(OH)D, from which the active 1,25(OH)D, is made as needed.

1,25(OH)D produced in the kidneys, and controlled by the parathyroid glands, is also a hormone. In the Vitamin D game, the hormone system, which affects the whole body, always wins. Working via the gut and bones, 1,25(OH)D controls the blood ionised calcium level. So in times of deficiency, other cells that need active Vitamin D for local use become vulnerable. The COVID-19 virus may have worked out that this includes your immune system. So you should too.

North of the equator where most of us live, UV light is completely blocked out by the atmosphere during winter. Now, at the time of the Equinox, unless we have been taking enough extra Vitamin D, our immune systems are surely at their weakest.

As the world goes into self-isolation, Vitamin D deficiency will get worse unless people take adequate supplements NOW. Any adult can safely take 100,000 Units of cholecalciferol as a single oral dose. Then immediately your liver will raise 25(OH) D to levels your immune system needs. No blood test is needed before this cheap, safe, and possibly life-saving move. So please go to your pharmacy now, do it, and tell your family and friends too.

It is hard to know what the effect of this simple dogmatic message was, but it has been circulated widely among professional friends, and posted on Facebook, and to date has nearly 3,000 'hits'. It brought home to many just how restricted access is to what we regard as decent doses of the 'Sunshine Vitamin' in the UK and USA.

Who we are

David Coussmaker Anderson

I was born on December 1st 1940. In 2018 I wrote and published an autobiography [Ref 1] which of course I strongly recommend. But this is not a promotional exercise, and what is relevant here is to explain a bit about how my mind works and has been working as I have tried to bring common sense into managing the pandemic.

I share with the late Dave Allen the claim to be a practicing atheist, although my origins were in moderate superstitious anglicanism rather than extreme punitive catholicism. From age 4 I knew I was going to be a doctor, and when at Rugby School I started to study biology at age 15 and learnt about evolution, I saw this as incompatible with special creation and the concept of an anthropocentric God. It took me a long time to come to the conclusion that what really matters is not what you believe, but what you do. I greatly enjoyed life as a doctor and I became a modestly successful endocrinologist, and Professor in Manchester, and then in 1991 in Hong Kong.

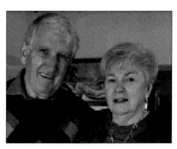

David & Jenny A

My interests in Medicine were, and remain broad. In fact, in Manchester I became increasingly frustrated with the confusion we were creating in the minds of future doctors, by allowing specialists to teach students things that their colleagues and fellow examiners (in other specialties) often didn't know. This seemed to be a recipe for confusion. It led me ultimately to make a series of clinical teaching films, *MediVision,* showing how specialists approached their own subject, and wherever possible demonstrating on live patients. My model was for teachers to watch these films with students in small groups, and so to update their own knowledge of other specialties in Medicine. Unfortunately this often conflicts with self-interest, academic ambition, and the need for senior academics to 'publish or be damned', which means having big departments full of research staff. When I made a film on Dog Bites and Rabies Prevention, I came to realise the power of enlightened self-interest often equates to maintaining said status, rather than to risk upsetting a powerful Committee Chairman. But as an outsider I felt that maybe it was up to me to stir up waves. There is no self-harm attached to telling the obvious truth outside your own field; and the only enemies you make aren't worth pleasing anyway.

After three years as Professor of Medicine in the Chinese University, and before I was pushed, I left official academic medicine. This seemed to happen to anyone there who stood up for truth. But I stayed on in Hong Kong and moved into private practice while continuing to make *MediVision* films. Then in 2008 I retired from Medicine altogether, or so I thought, and moved with my wife Jenny to Umbria. We feel extremely privileged in retirement, still being healthy and having active minds. And as we both have pensions, for the first time we are paid the same whether we work or not. This transition allowed me to pursue interests and obsessions outside Medicine. Thus, between 2000 and 2020 I have pursued the following;

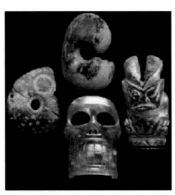

Hongshan artefacts: Jade pig-dragon; Jade Zhu; Agate cow god; Meteoritic glass skull mask

- Collecting and studying Neolithic jade, agate and other carvings from the Northern Chinese Hongshan Culture which dates back at least 10,000 years, and is being systematically and wilfully destroyed under the eyes of the Chinese authorities. I have written an illustrated book on Hongshan Jade Treasures. [Ref 2]

- I have fought against injustice and for reform of the global criminal justice system, in Italy and the USA, and co-authored a book on malicious prosecutions, including that of Amanda Knox and her then boyfriend in Italy. [Ref 3]

- I find myself seriously questioning the accepted model of climate change and global warming, and exploring a less convenient alternative, namely Jet Stream Abuse by high-flying commercial aircraft. There is currently an opportunity to explore that, once planes start flying again, which I fear will not be taken!

- I have undertaken extensive field work on a meteorite impact in Northern China and the destruction of a global human civilisation between 12,800 and 11,600 years ago.

- And I think I have sorted out the mystery of Malta's Cart ruts, which probably date back to the above lost civilisation, and which I postulate were used for aquaponic culture.

This has all been a fascinating by-product of being a Professor in Medicine who defied what was expected, by not being over-specialised. This life as a jack of all trades is all too often equated with being master of none, although 200 years ago it might have earned the more complimentary epithet of 'Renaissance Man'. Back then I feel my co-author and I would have been derided for arguing against bleeding people to death. We thought all that had ended, and that we are now gloriously

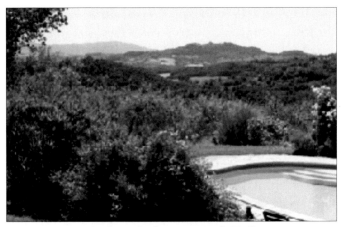

Umbria, looking towards Todi

and scientifically enlightened. And then Coronavirus came along and exploited a defect in collective human behaviour, revealing herd thinking (or non-thinking) and a singular unwillingness to confront the obvious, but testing us to death instead.

So we now fast forward to early 2020, and rumour spreads from Wuhan in central China of a new epidemic with a new coronavirus, believed as with SARS-1 in 2003 to have come from a wild animal sold in China's disgusting so-called 'wet markets'. In January and February in Italy, as this disaster hit Europe, I was concentrating on my putative 12,800 years BP meteorite impact, and planning a trip back to Inner Mongolia for one last time, when I started to wake up. I tend to have my best ideas while dreaming in the early morning hours. The first thing I awoke to is that the virus uses the ACE2 receptor to gain entry to the epithelial cells. There was some suggestion that the elderly with high blood pressure treated with an ACE inhibitor might be especially susceptible to this virus or maybe even be protected. In fact this prompted me to contact an old Hong Kong Colleague and friend, Prof Brian Tomlinson who put me right on some of the details. The main thing is that this virus gains entry to cells by latching onto these surface receptors, and the active form of Vitamin D3, 1,25(OH)D (calcitriol) blocks this receptor.

Then on around March 18th the connection with Vitamin D-deficiency suddenly hit me, Nebuchadnezzar-like, at around 4.30 a.m, and I got up and started to read up about Vitamin D and respiratory tract infections. One thing this pandemic has brought home is the power of getting information from the internet. And this even includes powerful, published, peer-reviewed unassailable analyses. Of course this did not include randomised controlled clinical trials on Covid-19, but then a pilot doesn't get that luxury either when he goes into free-fall, as the world suddenly was. It was this flash, and the upcoming spring Equinox (March 21st) that prompted me, helped by my wife, to make the short film described above.

David Stuart Grimes

I was born on November 26th 1943, in what is now the Royal Salford Hospital, where almost four decades later my co-author became Professor of Endocrinology. I was brought up in Prestwich, north Manchester into a Methodist family that was open to thought, and light on dogma. I am now what might be called an apatheist, in that I am not really interested in the sterile argument as to whether or not God exists. I went to Stand Grammar School in Whitefield, where I was fortunate in having what in retrospect was a standard but good education.

I went on to study Medicine at Manchester University. Medicine is not 'read' but studied in real life and death, and so is much more interesting and demanding. University and hospital education back then gave huge opportunities for learning, but today medical education seems grossly over-structured. We learned about things we might never see, but the knowledge was never wasted. We each had to deliver 20 babies, but I have done no such thing since, by good fortune not even my own three. It could be said that my paternal responsibilities ended with the conceptions, but even though my working hours turned out to be very long I was not an entirely absent father.

After qualification in 1966 I worked in the Manchester Royal Infirmary, and in 1968, shortly after I married my wonderful wife Jenny, I became the Resident Medical Officer. This was a post with considerable responsibility for all medical emergency admissions. The working

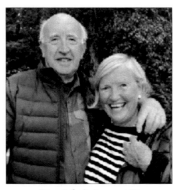

David & Jenny G

time was unimaginable today, being on duty every weekday, plus alternate nights and alternate weekends. It gave me a great deal of clinical experience, never to be forgotten. Boxing Day in December 1968 saw the onset of the epidemic of Hong Kong flu. There was no warning and no preparation, even though it was an international pandemic. I remember well the large number of medical emergency admissions (displacing elective surgical activity) and the deaths, reported as 80,000 in the UK.

It is difficult to imagine now, but in those days there were no intensive care units and no personal protective equipment.

I completed my broad-based post-graduate training in London and Manchester and ultimately was appointed as consultant physician and gastro-enterologist with the East Lancashire Hospitals Trust, based in Blackburn and later also in Burnley. I had excellent colleagues with forty happy and productive years, finishing my hospital work at the age of 70. Later in my working life I became the consultant physician with the Lancashire and South Cumbria Chronic Fatigue Syndrome Service. This seems to be strange but I had always tried to be helpful and no other consultant would take on this role. I had not been specifically 'trained' for this (there were no trainers) but found it to be the most challenging and rewarding work that I had done. It was purely clinical with very minimal use of blood tests and imaging. Contrary to medical and public opinion, I was convinced that I was dealing with real physical disease, but I had to think out for myself a biomedical model on which I could develop my understanding and my clinical work (conceptual models are essential to applied understanding, as we shall see later in our story). I felt that the patients were suffering from down-regulation of mitochondrial function, like hibernation but not reversible.

As with the understanding of Vitamin D in relation to immunity and the response (or non-response) to the pandemic of Covid-19, it was vital to bring together the clinical aspects of the disease and the basic biochemical research of which most medical doctors are totally unaware. Patients with chronic fatigues syndromes (the plural is deliberate) frequently had a fascinating maternal

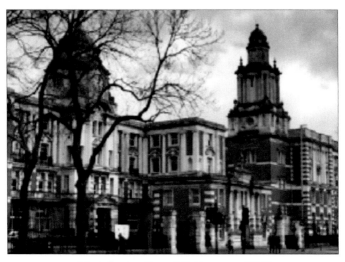
Manchester Royal Infirmary, 1975

family thread, pointing towards an inherited mitochondria tendency that was not always expressed in clinical illness. It was unfortunately a 'Cinderella' service in which the NHS was not interested, and much to my disappointment and that of the patients and their families, it was closed down. The clinical experience stimulated an interest in mitochondrial function and bio-energetics, that continues to this day.

The gastroenterology work was busy but straight-forward. My main challenge became to understand why the residents of Blackburn and the cities of the north-west of England, and especially the south Asian ethnic minority, had a such a bad health profile. The usual simplistic explanation was 'lifestyleism', that they were architects of their own health disadvantage. Such victim-blaming was convenient to the Government, which could then absolve itself of responsibility. But published evidence showed that it was false to blame the victims. Unfortunately, published information is usually 'untouched by human brain', as suggested by my mentor the remarkable 'Teddy' Chester, Professor of Social Administration at Manchester University.

This took me on a long research journey into the seriously underestimated importance of Vitamin D deficiency in the geography of disease and personal susceptibility. The realisation that Vitamin D and cholesterol had the same precursor chemical (7-dehydrocholesterol) led me to wonder if there was close metabolic connection. Although this turned out not to be the case it led me further into an interest in 'cholesterol'. It became clear to me that the diet-cholesterol-heart hypothesis is completely bogus, but with many vested interests, and we will see more of these later in our story. I realised that the high mortality form of coronary heart disease was the most serious epidemic, even pandemic, of the 20th century (about 400 million deaths), and that it might have been the result of a micro-organism, the identity of which has never been seriously investigated. Like all epidemics it had what were very well recorded features, namely an onset (about 1926), a peak (about 1970), and an end, in the second decade of the 21st century. Vitamin D was important because although its deficiency was not the cause of coronary heart disease it was the major determinant of its social and physical geography. These studies led to the award of MD in 1993, and the publication a book 'Vitamin D and Cholesterol: the importance of the Sun' in 2009. [Ref 4]

My research ran alongside my clinical work in East Lancashire, an area where I had a great interest in the industrial history and heritage. My other hospital duties were as Medical Director of the Trust for ten years, and also involvement in education within the north-west region, including medical management training.

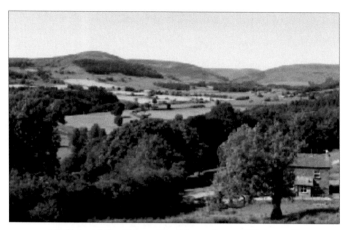

Valley of the River Hodder, above Whitewell

I live in Langho, and as I look north from my house across the beautiful Ribble Valley, past Stonyhurst College, and into the almost hidden Hodder Valley, I see a summit at 1,000 feet above sea level. It is Browsholme Heights, above Browsholme Hall and the delightful Inn at Whitewell. It was at Browsholme Heights that the Alston branch of my family were farmers in 1750 and subsequently. I have therefore not come far in life, but it has been a rewarding journey.

Having continued through my Blog [Ref 5] my interest in epidemics, and the geography and ethnicity of disease, my interest was immediately attracted to the pandemic of Covid-19. Knowing the extent of Vitamin D deficiency of the South Asian community (90%) and of the general population (74%) within Blackburn, I realised how important would be the use of Vitamin D in protecting them and the population of the nation against this new virus. This fell mainly but not completely upon stony ground.

Healthcare in Italy and Great Britain

David Anderson

One great advantage of living in Italy as we Andersons now do, is that health care provision here is much less 'Nanny-fied' than in the UK. We left Britain for Hong Kong in 1991, since when things seem to have lapsed into 'Medicine by Numbers', under a do-gooder organisation called 'NICE' (The 'National Institute for Clinical Excellence'). I have long been surprised and appalled by just how restricted and restrictive pharmacies in the UK have become, in comparison with a much more *laissez faire* attitude in Italy. I am known by our local pharmacy to be a doctor, and so can buy any common antibiotic without a doctor's prescription. I once tried that in London for my wife who had a urinary tract infection, but I had stopped paying to stay on the UK Medical Register so it didn't work – I had to get a prescription, which I eventually got from a German Doctor Hess in a clinic based in a nearby hospital, after pulling rank on the West Indian sister-in-charge. Three hours later, I returned to the pharmacy with the nice said prescription, and got the antibiotic free of charge to me, but not of course to the NHS.

But returning to Vitamin D, in the UK it is controlled by a Scientific Advisory Committee on Nutrition (SACN), which in 2016 published its Guidelines on Vitamin D. This is now seen as being set in tablets of stone. it seems that in Italy there is no 'NICE' Committee to decide how much of this essential sunshine Vitamin D is good for me. So anyone can go into a pharmacy, as I have done for years and buy small bottles containing 100,000 units of Vitamin D3 (which is in fact a mere 2.5 mg) for consumption every 2 or 3 months over the winter, cost around 6 Euros. But when I made enquiries of one of the manufacturers, Abiogen, which is based in Pisa, I found that they also marketed it in vials of the same dose in 1ml of olive oil, 'for intramuscular or oral use' in boxes of 6, cost 4 Euros a box. Since then, with the cooperation of Gianni the pharmacist I have obtained three consignments of 200 to 600 vials of Vitamin D in olive oil. I gave 200 to the local hospital for distribution to Covid-19 Unit staff, who greatly appreciated it. And then when doctors in the UK, mainly of African or Asian origin started to die from Covid-19, [Ref 6] on March 25th. I contacted by email the fellow-endocrinologist Professor Parag Singhal of Weston Super Mare, who is also Hon Secretary of the organisation British Association of Physicians of Indian Origin (BAPIO). Since then I have sent by courier service 900 vials for distribution to his members. We have had no complaints.

Dr John O'Driscoll is a good friend based in Manchester, who 40 years ago worked with me in Hope (now called Royal Salford) Hospital, when I was particularly interested in Paget's Disease of Bone. Two of his three children work in the front-line, and both contracted coronavirus, fortunately heeding my advice on Vitamin D3, which had to be bought via the internet in capsules of 5000 units. Manchester is the location of one of the Florence Nightingale Hospitals, designed to take 1000 patients, but in fact never used; on John's advice I contacted the man in charge, Professor Tony Redmond (once a colleague at Hope), with an offer to send 1,200 vials of 100,000 units each, to be distributed to staff. He thanked me but said he would have to put it to his committee. They in their (lack of) wisdom turned it down on the grounds that it would need a Randomised

Controlled Trial (RCT) first! So this Committee refused to give to Frontline Health Care Workers a vitamin that at worst could do no harm! We will return later to consider the nature of evidence, the value of observational studies, the place of RCT's, Meta-analysis, and Reason. We challenge anyone reading this book to cite any example of harm that has come from any adult taking a single dose of 100,000IU of Vitamin D.

Hormones, Immunity and Vitamin D

Evolutionary History of Vitamin D

For more than a billion years animal life has been able to synthesise squalene, a long molecular chain composed of 30 carbon atoms and 50 hydrogen atoms. Then aquatic animal life acquired an enzyme that caused this molecule to establish intramolecular bonds to create a 4-ring structure, called 7-dehydrocholesterol (7-DHC), from

Squalene

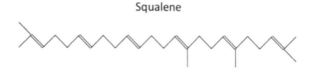

7-dehydrocholesterol (7-DHC)

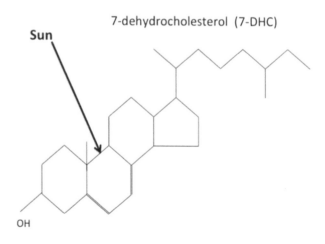

which cholesterol and steroid hormones are produced (one metabolic step is the action of the enzyme HMG-CoA reductase that is blocked by statin drugs to reduce cholesterol synthesis). 7-DHC was initially formed by plankton, but it was so fundamental to life that throughout evolution that it was adopted as essential by all advanced animal life-forms.

UV sunlight of a specific wavelength (UVB, 280–315nm) can split a specific bond within the 7-DHC molecule to form pre-Vitamin D3, which then spontaneously unfolds to become cholecalciferol (Vitamin D3). This is a physico-chemical reaction: there is no involvement of enzymes and strictly speaking it is not 'synthesis', which is a biochemical process. The reaction absorbs the energy of the UV light and thus diminishes the UV energy that might otherwise have damaged the living tissues. [Ref 6]

Vitamin D - Cholecalciferol

Vitamin D production

(Unless specified from now on we will use the designation 'Vitamin D' to refer to D3, cholecalciferol, which is the form made by animals).

In humans Vitamin D is immediately absorbed into the blood-stream, and carried mainly protein-bound to the liver. In furry mammals, 7-DHC is secreted on to the surface of the skin in the oils that provide water-proofing. Sunlight (UVB) converts 7-DHC into vitamin D, which the animal will then swallow when licking its fur. In the sea, plankton are eaten by small fish, and small fish are eaten by larger ones. Vitamin D from fish also becomes part of the food chain which will reach humans.

Fungi synthesise ergosterol rather than 7-dehydro-cholesterol, and when exposed to UV light Vitamin D2 (ergocalciferol) is produced. When we ingest fungi, this D2 is absorbed and enters the same metabolic pathways as cholecalciferol; but it is certainly different and has a shorter half-life than the D3 we make in our skin under the action of UVB.

Vitamin D activation

Vitamin D itself is inert. As blood circulates through the liver, it is hydroxylated to 25(OH)D (calcidiol). It then becomes a pre-hormone and strictly speaking it is no longer a vitamin. 25(OH)D, the storage form, is stable and returns to the blood where it is largely bound to a 25(OH)D-specific binding-protein (DBP), or by the general purpose protein albumin; some is also stored in body fat, the quantity being increased in obese individuals. 25(OH) D in blood plasma constitutes the reservoir available for instant use by the cells of body tissues. Activation is

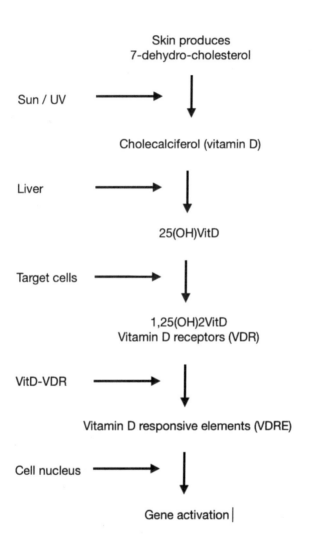

Skin produces
7-dehydro-cholesterol

Sun / UV ⟶ ↓

Cholecalciferol (vitamin D)

Liver ⟶ ↓

25(OH)VitD

Target cells ⟶ ↓

1,25(OH)2VitD
Vitamin D receptors (VDR)

VitD-VDR ⟶ ↓

Vitamin D responsive elements (VDRE)

Cell nucleus ⟶ ↓

Gene activation

achieved by the addition of another hydroxyl group, in the 1 position of the molecule to form 1,25(OH)D, or (calcitriol). This is the chemical messenger designed to switch on a wide range of metabolic processes, most of which involve calcium transport. One important site for this is in the kidneys. The other major site is in the cells that are responsible for immunity.

Vitamin D and the endocrine control of blood ionised calcium

The relevant endocrine system works as follows; the parathyroid glands in the neck monitor the blood ionised calcium level, and if it dips too low they secrete their hormone, PTH, which travels in the blood and acts on cells in the kidneys. Acting via cell surface receptors and cyclic AMP, they induce the enzyme 1-alpha hydroxylase, which converts 25(OH)D to 1,25(OH)D. This travels as a hormone in the blood to promote calcium absorption across the gut and if necessary from bone, which is the main internal store of calcium and phosphate. The rise in serum calcium switches off PTH secretion, in a classical negative feedback loop. This is the most obvious role of Vitamin D and its metabolites, and as it was the first to be worked out, as well as the greediest, it still dominates the thinking of most nutritionists and endocrinologists. Dangerously and illogically they have used these needs to dictate what they believe the whole body needs.

It is as if in a famine, only the adult males are considered; pregnant women and children are left to starve, and food supplies are calculated accordingly.

Vitamin D's action at the cellular level

Once the mechanisms at the blood level were worked out, attention was directed to changes in cells. 1,25(OH)D binds to a (specific) Vitamin D receptor (VDR). Vitamin A1 (retinol) is also important, and its receptor (RXR) forms a complex with VDR, and the pair together switch on a multitude of specific genes in target tissues. The above system also acts locally, below the 'endocrine radar', in very many tissues in the body, including the immune system. It can do so because of locally produced enzyme 1-alpha hydroxylase, needed to make 1,25(OH)D for the same cell or the one next door. But only if there is enough 25(OH)D. In case of shortage of 25(OH)D, the endocrine role always dominates because of the over-riding need to control circulating calcium. It follows that in cases of Vitamin D deficiency all other systems that need 25(OH)D play second fiddle to these endocrine requirements. It is therefore entirely predictable that those systems least able to fight for themselves have the greatest need for a powerful advocate for higher 25(OH)D levels. This is a concept fundamental to understanding what has gone wrong in the coronavirus pandemic.

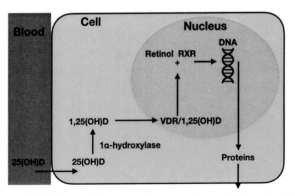

Intracellular and intranuclear actions of Vitamin D

Immunity and the role of Vitamin D

Key cells in defensive immunity are the macrophages ('big eateres') which can eat bacteria, the lymphocytes, and dendritic cells, and they all depend on having access to Vitamin D. There are two types of lymphocyte. B-lymphocytes (derived from the Bursa of Fabricius) produce antibodies, while T-lymphocytes (derived from the Thymus) are concerned with cellular immunity. But there is also a basic immunity against new and unknown invaders, and this provides immune surveillance day by day, and escalates in response to a serious infection. This activation has been researched in great detail during the past few decades, and is critically dependent on having 25(OH)D levels well above the minimum needed by the body's (greedy) circulating endocrine needs. Important Committee members, please pay special attention!

The seasons, rickets, industrialisation and the discovery of vitamin D

Those who ignore history are destined to repeat it, so politicians please also pay attention. The seasons are driven by the 23.5-degree axis of rotation of the earth relative to its rotation round the sun. This tilt doesn't matter much around the equator. But as our species moved in large numbers progressively northwards away from the equator, UVB deficiency and therefore winter Vitamin D deficiency became progressively more extreme. As a result we progressively lost out natural melanin sunblock: pale-skinned mutants had a considerable survival advantage.

The industrial revolution, which started in Britain, led to a massive movement of people away from the countryside into ever-growing cities. Steam-driven

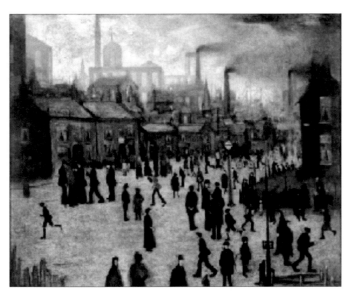

A manufacturing town – L S Lowry

factories were built with the workers living close by in small terraced houses or apartment blocks, in Glasgow called tenements. Coal-fired domestic heating, steam trains, serious atmospheric pollution, long factory hours for men, women and children, all meant there was very little exposure to the sun. In this environment, many children were found to have a new disease, rickets [Ref 7]. The rachitic or 'rickety' children were also noted to be 'sickly'. Glasgow was the rickets capital of the world, but improvement occurred when rachitic children were sent to live with family members in their traditional coastal villages, with clean air and with plenty of fish to eat. Likewise in Austria rickets and general illness appeared in the factory children, and improvement occurred when, like Heidi, they were sent to families in the farms in the mountains.

So it was in Glasgow and Austria that the importance of the sun and fish oil were recognised, and the vital ingredient was later identified as Vitamin D. The key publications were obviously well before the modern era and Randomised Controlled Trials (RCTs). Careful observation led to understanding, and implementation followed and gradually brought rickets to an end. It was also noted that families that had children with rickets often also had others with 'consumption', which we now know to have been tuberculosis. With movement to the coast or the mountains, both rickets and tuberculosis improved.

Critical observations by a Scottish physician in Bombay

A particularly interesting and relevant study took place when a Scottish physician, Dr HS Hutchison visited the Civil Hospital in Nasik, in Bombay (now Mumbai), India. [Ref 8] With his assistant SJ Shah he investigated the prevalence of disease in the local population and found that once again rickets and tuberculosis co-existed in the same families. However, in total contrast to Glasgow, this occurred in the wealthy families. He realised that in India poor people spent their days outside working in the fields, whereas the wealthy were able stay indoors out of the sun, and the women were able to practise purdah. This study was decisive in linking rickets and tuberculosis together, and both to Vitamin D.

Heliotherapy: treatment with sunlight and UV

The curing of rickets became straightforward. It was clearly a direct consequence of Vitamin D deficiency; but tuberculosis was more difficult. In 1882 the German pathologist Robert Koch showed conclusively that tuberculosis is due a bacterium, subsequently called *Mycobacterium tuberculosis*. If tuberculosis was caused by a micro-organism, what was the role of sunlight and Vitamin D?

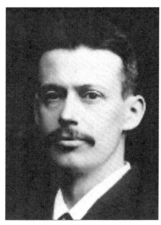

Niels Ryberg Finsen

Niels Ryberg Finsen was born in the Faroe Islands in 1860 and received his medical education in Denmark. He showed that tuberculosis of the skin (Lupus vulgaris) could be cured by UV light, and for this he received the Nobel Prize for Medicine in 1903. He felt that UV light was having a systemic effect, thereby improving the internal heath of his patients, but he was unable to investigate this further. His health had been impaired for many years by constrictive pericarditis, thought to be caused by hydatid disease acquired from sheep droppings in childhood. It led to his early death at the age of 44, just one year after he received his Nobel Prize. Finsen's work was very influential.

The Heliotherapy (treatment by the sun), and sanatorium movement developed in the early years of the 20th century. [Ref 9] There was no specific treatment for tuberculosis at the time, but the clean air helped, especially at high altitudes in Switzerland. It was clear that sunlight was improving the body's defensive system, but the mechanisms were not understood and the word 'immunity' was still in the future.

Cod liver oil and heliotherapy for 'Consumption'

If the sun was helping in the treatment of tuberculosis, was it acting via Vitamin D? A remarkable clinical trial took place at The Hospital for Consumption (later the Brompton Hospital) in London in 1848, and it has been described by Professor Malcolm Green [Ref 10]. Vitamin D had not yet been identified, but cod liver oil was given as an empirical treatment. 542 patients were given standard treatment and 535 patients were given cod liver oil in addition. In 5.6% of the control subjects (not given cod liver oil) the disease was 'arrested' while 33.3% died. In those given cod liver oil, the disease was arrested in 18.1% and only 18.8% died. This controlled study demonstrated a considerable benefit from cod liver oil, but it was many years before Vitamin D was identified as the active ingredient.

Heliotherapy continued until the late 1950s when anti-tuberculosis antibiotics and chemotherapy came into use, but many older adults today remember 'sunshine clinics' of their childhood, in which they and other children would sit wearing knickers and goggles in a circle around a UV lamp.

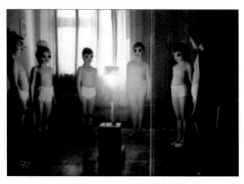

"Sunshine clinic" UK c1969

Vitamin D and defensive immunity

In response to infection the genes of the T-lymphocytes do two things. First, they produce defensive inflammatory proteins called cytokines, that kill bacteria and viruses (other cells also produce cytokines). Second, the genes are stimulated to produce additional VDRs. This becomes a positive feedback loop, producing escalation of the defensive immune response, in some respects by a factor of up to 75 times. This is potentially very powerful, but there is a snag. The additional VDRs cannot become active without more 1,25(OH)D molecules. VDR is synthesised within the cell, but human cells can only make 1,25(OH)D from its substrate 25(OH)D, which comes from the blood, and its formation has been described. If the Vitamin D (as 25(OH)D) level in the blood is low or lacking altogether, protective escalation cannot proceed. A blood level of Vitamin D greater than 30ng/ml (75nmol/L) is absolutely essential to provide adequate amounts of 25(OH)D to escalate defence against serious and potentially life-threatening infection. [Ref 11] There is no excuse for not measuring 25(OH)D levels, as assays are freely available and inexpensive.

Vitamin D and protection against the cytokine storm

During the pandemic of Covid-19 there have been reports of a 'cytokine storm' preceding critical illness and death. What does this mean? It is effectively an uncontrolled inflammatory response. But why the lack of control? Its main features are serious clinical deterioration plus a very high level of C-reactive protein (CRP) in the blood, which has also been noted to be associated with a low blood level of Vitamin D. So what is going on here?

Inflammation is a defensive process designed to destroy invading micro-organisms. The process is first associated with the production of Tumour Necrosis Factor alpha (TNFα), and the final steps and restoration to normal, with a transition to Transforming Growth Factor beta (TGFβ).[Ref 12]. The 1,25(OH)D-VDR/RXR complex controls the switch. If TNFα remains dominant, a cytokine storm will occur, but if the 25(OH)D reserve in the blood is sufficient, the above complex will reduce TNFα [Ref 13] and switch to TGFβ domination, with successful resolution of inflammation. This regulation is only possible if there is enough 25(OH)D in the blood plasma reservoir.

Actions of Vitamin D on other organs

In addition to the above calcium/endocrine and immune systems, cells of the following organs and tissues are also able to hydroxylate 25(OH)D to 1,25(OH)D, and make VDRs: parathyroid glands, dendritic cells, prostate, colon, vascular endothelium, bone, brain (basal ganglia, cerebellum and cortex), skin, lymph nodes, placenta, breast, thyroid, and chondrocytes. The functions of 1,25(OH)D in these tissues are not always clear, but activation of many genes has been recognised.

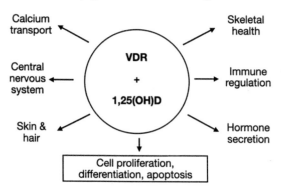

It is likely that vitamin D is the key that unlocks many intracellular and genetic processes. There is much research to be done, with very great potential benefit.

Current Committee obsessions with risks of toxicity

Unfortunately, in the UK the Scientific Advisory Committee on Nutrition (SACN) is obsessed with the very rare Vitamin D toxicity, despite case reports indicating that usually this is the result of medication errors. Very rarely it can result from active tuberculosis, or the related disorder sarcoidosis, in which macrophages overproduce 1,25(OH)D locally. SACN members have not understood the implications of a need for an increased requirement of Vitamin D at times of serious infection. So not knowing better, they set requirements for D3 supplements at the minimum needed to prevent rickets and osteomalacia, and conserve bone health. Furthermore SACN recommendations have become set in tablets of stone as the vitamin D subcommittee was disbanded in 2016, and people able best to serve as champions of higher levels seem to be dying out. In this era of obligatory Peer Review, whose responsibility is it to review a Peerless Panel of one's Peers? Is it really a question of safety in numbers, or is science also important?

We are each (identical twins aside) unique in our own special mix of genes. This brings with it a great deal of variation in requirements, responses and propensities to disease. For Vitamin D this also applies to individual tissues. Nature knows this, and with Vitamin D and the unpredictability of sunshine, has built in a large margin of safety. As two lifelong clinicians born with reasonable brains and ideation, this was what used to be most interesting and motivating about clinical practice, and clinical research. Unfortunately, as with much of modern clinical medicine, logic, common sense, and use of the individual doctor's brain to help the individual patient has given place to dictat by Committee that acts as though it knows all the answers.

Dr Edward de Bono said that the greatest bar to progress is the need to be right all the time. 'It is better to have enough ideas for some of them to be wrong, than to always be right by having no ideas at all.' If this is extended to rule by Committee, the loudest voice and the lowest denominator of thought will always win, and this is both ubiquitous and dangerous.

Considerations of Ethnicity

Variations of vitamin D production with ethnicity and location

Humankind first evolved in tropical Africa, living as a hunter-gatherer with the days spent outside and clothing minimal or absent. The sun in the tropics is high enough to produce vitamin D all the year round. But over 100,000 years much of our species has migrated to more temperate zones of the planet where there are exaggerated seasons.

The more atmosphere that sunlight must pass through, the greater is the amount of UV light that is blocked. As a general rule, when a person's shadow is longer than their height, when the sun is at declination of more than 45 degrees from the vertical, there will not be enough UVB light close to sea level to split the 7-DHC molecule, so no Vitamin D will be formed. The further from the equator, the longer will be the winter season without Vitamin D production. The greater the altitude, the thinner is the atmosphere, and so the greater is the Vitamin D production.

The effect of skin colour on Vitamin D production

A paler skin had the advantage at places distant from the equator that it is more efficient at producing Vitamin D. Twenty minutes of white skin in the same sun will produce the same amount of Vitamin D as 120 minutes for very dark skin. The skin pigment melanin absorbs UV energy, and less is available for breaking the critical bond in 7-DHC. Survival depended on an adequate supply of Vitamin D production in the skin. An exception is the Inuit people of the sub-Arctic region of North America and Greenland, whose diet was almost exclusively of oily fish, containing large quantities of vitamin D, from the action of the sun on plankton. During the 20th century Inuit people had unfortunate dealings with so-called 'civilisation'. They changed to a 'western diet' and their health deteriorated considerably, with the inevitable dramatic reduction of dietary Vitamin D.

North-west Europe is unusual in being heavily populated but lying on the same latitude as Hudson Bay in Canada, and Siberia. The Gulf Stream brings warm water from the Central Atlantic Ocean. As north-west Europe is so far from the equator, Vitamin D can be produced for only four to six months of the year. The very pale skin of the Scandinavian people in particular has been the result of evolutionary natural selection. Also, the seas around Scandinavia have been rich in fish and the people have enjoyed a fish-rich diet to provide additional vitamin D.

Ethnicity and vitamin D

Living in the tropics and spending time outdoors is the best way to enjoy a good supply of Vitamin D, and the blood levels of such people should give a guide to the ideal. The Maasai and Hadzabe people of East Africa have respectively average blood vitamin D levels of 47.6 and 43.6 ng/ml (119 and 109 nmol/L) [Ref 14]. So it would appear that we should have a target blood level of about 40ng/ml (100 nmol/L), as this is what evolution and nature decided.

A problem arises when pastoral life in tropical Africa is disrupted by 'civilisation', including religion, and in many areas driven historically by the slave trade. The results are excessive clothing, indoor life, and most of all, emigration to temperate zones, usually entailing city rather than rural life. This is not the result of evolution and the disadvantages are serious.

Research undertaken a number of years ago by one of the authors (DSG) showed the vitamin D status of people living in the north-west of England, and especially those whose families moved from South Asia. 1574 people with a South Asian ethnicity had a median blood vitamin D level of 9.8ng/ml (22nmol/L), meaning that half had a level less than this. 600 (38%) had a level between the recommended minimum of 10ng/ml (25nmol/L) and 30 ng/ml, meaning that they were deficient. Only 60 (3.8%) had a level greater than 30ng/ml (75nmol/L), which is an acceptable minimum. The 815 white controls had a median level of 18ng/ml, twice that of the ethnic Asian group, but still low. Only 107 (13%) had blood levels of vitamin D greater than 30ng/ml. This shows how precarious are the vitamin D reserves in the great majority of people in north-west England, especially in those of South Asian ethnicity.

In the following two illustrations, each vertical column represents an individual person in the study. The height of the column is determined by the blood level of vitamin D. The horizontal red line is the minimum threshold of the ideal range of vitamin D. The vertical orange line is the middle of the range, the median. The horizontal yellow line shows the Vitamin D level of that divides the highest half and the lowest half.

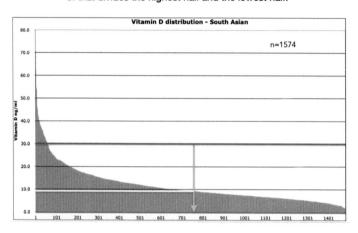

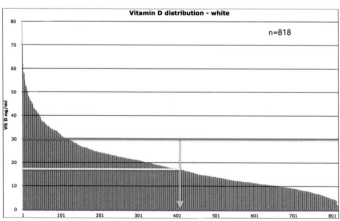

Pandemics Past and Present

Historical Pandemics

Epidemics, now called pandemics if all continents are affected simultaneously, are not new. In the Bible we can read about plagues without fully understanding them. Then there was the Plague of Justinian in the 6th century. But the Black Death of the 14th century, caused by the rat flea-borne bacterium *Yersinia pestis*, is better documented, with total deaths estimated at up to 200 million, perhaps a quarter of the Western population. In England we had the Great Plague of London in 1665/66, with deaths in excess of 100,000. This time it was brought to an end by the Great Fire of London, which killed all the rats and the infected fleas that they carried. During the 19th century there was a series of epidemics of cholera, with about 25,000 deaths in the UK, but 2 million deaths in Russia and many million in India. The classical epidemiological study of Dr John Snow in London linked the 1854 epidemic to a contaminated water supply. The disease in Europe was brought to an end by the understanding encapsulated by the Germ Theory of disease, and realisation of the vital of importance of keeping human waste well away from supplies of drinking-water.

Immediately following World War 1, during 1918/19, the population of Europe and much of the world experienced the pandemic of Spanish Flu, so called because one of the first dignitaries to be affected was King Alfonso XIII of Spain. It led to the deaths of more

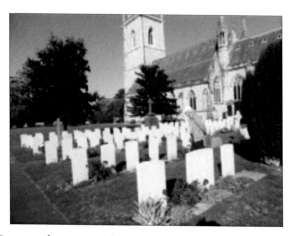

*Graves of young soldiers (mainly Canadian) who died
from Spanish flu, 1919.
Bodelwyddan Marble Church, North Wales*

than 50 million people world-wide, including 228,000
in Britain. The next 20th century pandemic was Asian
Flu in 1957/58, caused by the influenza A virus H2N2,
and which originated in Guizhou, China. This killed
more than 2 million people world-wide, including 30,000
in the UK. In 1968/69 we experienced the pandemic of
Hong Kong flu, with about 4 million deaths world-wide
and an estimated 80,000 in the UK. The SARS epidemic
of 2003 caused a mere 8,098 reported cases and 774
deaths worldwide; it was contained by good public health
measures and contact tracing in Hong Kong and after
some delay in China.

It might have been expected that with this history of
epidemics, our nation would have prepared itself for
another, as being inevitable; yet this did not happen. The
UK government undertook Exercise Cygnus in 2016, the
purpose being to plan for a 'flu' epidemic in the future.

By 'flu' is meant a highly transmissible virus infection acting via the respiratory tract, and having a significant mortality rate especially among the elderly. The scenario of Cygnus was an epidemic that in the UK would cause up to 400,000 excess deaths. This was an extravagant hypothetical number, twice the number of UK deaths from Spanish Flu. It was leaked that the exercise identified serious failings in the UK to deal with such an epidemic, but the report has never been published.

The pandemic of Covid-19

There is a strong tendency for viral epidemics and pandemics to occur towards the end of winter in the Northern hemisphere where most of the world's population lives. Although you would not have guessed it from the Press or Politicians, there is a mass of evidence that this is because our innate immune defence system is dependent on adequate levels of the 'Sunshine Vitamin', D3, which is only formed during the summer months, and then only in individuals with enough exposure to the midday sun and so to UVB radiation. This innate defence system has been ignored in this pandemic, for reasons discussed later. In fact it can reasonably be argued that it has been due to the interface of two pandemics – one a virus, one seasonal D-deficiency- amplified by uncontrolled global air travel.

On December 31st 2019 Wuhan Municipal Health Commission, China, reported a cluster of cases of an unusual form of pneumonia in the polluted city of Wuhan, Hubei Province. A novel virus was eventually identified to be corona in type. This is the same family responsible for SARS and MERS, as well as being implicated in 4 versions of the common or garden common cold. It was stated that the virus had originated in bats and had jumped a species boundary into humankind in the wet market in Wuhan. It is, however, risky to take anything official coming out of China at face value, and there was initially an undoubted attempt to suppress information. Thus a doctor (who subsequently died of the infection) tried to speak out, and was arrested for spreading false rumours. China released the genetic sequence of what was called Covid-19, on January 12th 2020 (Covid = corona virus infection disease, and 19 refers to the year of recognition). On the following day the first case outside China was recorded in Thailand. By January 30th there were cases reported in another 17 countries.

It is doubtful if the seriousness of the impending situation was appreciated as the UK Government led by Prime Minister Boris Johnson, was preoccupied by 'Brexit Day' on January 31st. Covid-19 first struck Europe with devastating results in Northern Italy in February 2020. At the onset of the epidemic in the UK, the Secretary of State for Health, Matt Hancock, indicated in an interview with LBC that all the recommendations of the 2016 Cygnus exercise had been implemented, without explaining what they were.

By March 1st 2020 Italy had recorded 1694 cases and 34 deaths. The epidemic involved the Po valley and was centred on Bergamo. It soon became clear that this area had the worst air pollution in Europe, identified clearly on satellite images. Wuhan was also at the centre of an area of extreme air pollution, but the significance of these observations was not immediately obvious. Spain was the next European country to experience a large number of Covid-19 cases and deaths; at one point an ice rink was being used to store the dead. Air pollution was not significant in this instance, but of course atmospheric pollution restricts the passage of light through the air.

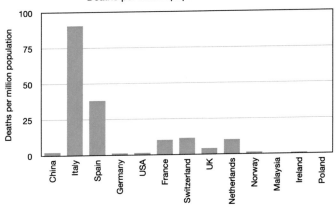

Deaths per million population March 23 2020

'Lockdown' was introduced in Italy on March 7th and in Spain on March 15th. By March 23rd Italy had experienced 90.5 deaths per million population and Spain half that. Lockdown is intended to protect the population by diminishing transmission between humans. On March 23rd the UK had experienced 284 deaths, 4.2 per million, and a decision was made to do likewise.

On April 23rd the deaths in Italy had risen to 429 per million, in Spain to 473 per million, and in the UK to 289 per million (19,507 total). There were even higher rates in Belgium (576 per million) and in tiny San Marino there were 39 deaths in a population of just 33,400. There was great variation, some countries such as Germany reporting a very large number of cases but relatively few deaths (64 per million on April 23rd). This was wrongly attributed to better hospital facilities in Germany. By the same reasoning, Russia must have by far the best hospital services: by mid-May, the UK had twice the number of cases per million than Russia, but 30 times the number of deaths per million! These variations were not easy to understand and it is futile to compare just two countries.

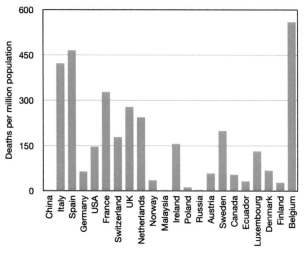

Deaths per million population April 23 2020

Mathematical advice, left to its own, as with Cygus, suggested that Covid-19 might infect 50 million of the 67.5 million UK population. If the mortality rate were to be 1% (not an unreasonable assumption) there would be 500,000 deaths, and the need for a vast number of intensive care beds. It would far exceed previous epidemics and the experiences of other countries subjected to the pandemic before the UK. However it gave a number against which anything less might be considered to be a political and medical success.

No other rational attempts were made to protect the population of the UK. Hospital services were redesigned and turned over almost entirely to Covid-19 patients, with considerable expansion of the number of intensive care beds. On the basis of the mathematical 'model' seven additional 'Nightingale' hospitals were developed with impressive speed and cost, but turned out to be unnecessary. A wasteful model, you might say. Apart from social distancing as part of the lockdown process, what else could be done to protect the public? Providing rescue services for the critically ill is not the same as preventing serious disease. There was no consideration of the importance of improving the human host defences rather than just concentrating on one virus. We and others failed in our attempts to bring this to national attention via the press or those in charge.

Epidemics eventually come to an end

Epidemics tend to run their course, for example Hong Kong Flu in 1968/69. At that time there was neither great publicity nor much international co-operation. There were no intensive care units, no personal protective equipment (PPE), no lockdown and no social distancing. Schools and workplaces remained open and transport continued. 80,000 deaths in the UK was a lot, but the epidemic still went away. If the death rate of those who were ill was 1%, we must assume that 8 million people were ill, most remaining at home. We have no idea how many people were infected as there was no RNA or even antibody testing available. The number infected in the UK could have been three times the number who were ill, in other words perhaps 25 million.

Once away, Hong Kong flu never came back. When an individual is infected by a bacterium or a virus, the body will mount a defensive immune response, the details of which will be explained later. If the individual does not die, the immune response to the specific micro-organism will be 'learned' with the formation of a specific clone of B-lymphocytes programmed to make a specific antibody. If a second infection occurs the defensive immunity from antibody production will be rapid and illness will at worst be mild.

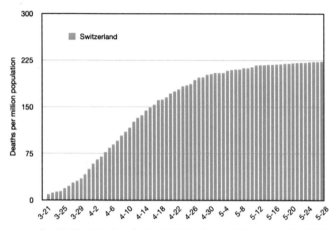

Corvid-19 epidemic in Switzerland. Deaths per million population (8.6M).
A steep rise and then during the second half of May, there were very few
deaths as the epidemic came to an end

Herd immunity

Once enough of the population have been infected and
so become resistant, (and the percentage depends on
the transmissibility of the virus), an epidemic will come
to an end. This is what is meant by 'herd immunity'.
Viruses do not go away but we become resistant through
acquired immunity to add to our inherited immunity. It is
sometimes stated that viruses mutate into a milder form.
Although this was a feature of 'The Andromeda Strain'
(author Michael Crichton, 1971), in real life it is only a
fiction.

Only the intrinsic immune system can be expected to
protect against a virus that is new to humankind, which
Covid-19 seems to be. The development of antibodies
follows, but takes time. So the main objective of the
response to a pandemic must be to maximise the innate
anti-viral resistance of the 67.5 million citizens of the UK,

and the billions world-wide. This is particularly important for people who appear to be at special risk of developing critical disease. Yet thus far efforts to enhance this anti-invasion system have not been on either the Government or the Private Industrial agenda. Instead all efforts are going into the development of a vaccine.

'The vaccine'

Vaccines provide immunity by exposing immunocytes (immunity cells) to critical parts of a virus or bacterium, which will induce antibodies without causing an illness. This takes time, and even longer to make certain that the vaccine is safe. This means that a vaccine will become available after the pandemic has come to an end, and perhaps only in 2021. It might then prevent a 'second wave', but there is another approach that was already available on March 23rd when lockdown was introduced in the UK. It was suggested one day earlier on DA's Youtube film. It is important to realise that a vaccine will provide defence against just one micro-organism, whereas Vitamin D activates defence against all micro-organisms.

UK Government 'action' – the mathematical approach

Since lockdown was introduced in the UK, the number of deaths has risen from 284 (4.2 per million) to 37,048 (548.9 per million) on May 27th, more than a hundred-fold increase. The prime minister has called this a success, and it is certainly substantially less than 500,000 deaths projected by the mathematicians. But how many fewer deaths would there have been if we had enhanced the innate immune responses of those who became critically ill and died?

The UK Government has been advised by its Scientific Advisory Group for Emergencies (SAGE). The membership of SAGE depends on the nature of the emergency. The pandemic of Covid-19 has resulted in SAGE having 57 members, two of whom do not want their names disclosed. The group is composed of mainly public health doctors, scientists, statisticians. A member who might have any knowledge of the enhancement of individual immunity is not obvious.

Statisticians emphasise the importance of the R number, the number of people to whom one infected person is likely to pass on the virus. R = 2 or more indicates an exponential spread. R = <1 indicates a much lower level of spread. But the important thing is surely how many of those infected will experience significant disease? It is the R number that drives the policy of lockdown.

Scientific reasoning and judgement

The process of scientific reasoning requires 'falsification'. It is easy to make a hypothesis, but in science it must be testable. At times of emergency, action might need to be taken on the basis of a plausible hypothesis. Judgement involves assessing the balance between potential benefit and potential harm. Implementation gives an opportunity to assess how robust the hypothesis might be. It is essential to ask the question 'Might I be wrong?'

Lockdown seemed at the time to be a sensible approach to protect the public. The isolation of Wuhan in China appears to have been successful within China, but failure to close down the airport allowed Covid-19 to be dispersed around the world. Lockdown has been implemented in many countries. Benefit is not obvious, as the more than a hundred-fold increase in deaths since lockdown in the UK indicates. And it has caused huge economic harm, the effects of which will last for many years to come. There is serious damage to schooling and universities, to the entertainment industry, restaurants, pubs, theatres, cinemas, holidays, air travel, and employment in general, although air quality has certainly improved greatly

The pandemic has affected Russia later than other European countries. The number of deaths has been low, on April 16th 233 (1.6 per million), but the number of cases high at 24,490 (168 per million). Despite this President Putin reversed the lockdown. Presumably he considered that the benefit was far from obvious but the economic damage was very serious. Italy and Spain also eased the lockdown. No nation has explicitly stated that lockdown has been of no tangible benefit, but only that the national epidemics would have been much worse without it, obviously a hypothetical view.

The key role of Imperial College, London

It seems that the policy to protect the population from death by Covid-19 was led by Professor Neil Ferguson of Imperial College, London University whose mathematical model was described as 'totally unreliable' and coding a 'buggy mess'.[1] Ferguson's previous predictions have been interesting. In 2002, He predicted up to 50,000 deaths from variant Creutzfeld-Jakob disease resulting from bovine spongiform encephalitis (BSE, or 'mad cow disease'). 178 people died. In 2005 he predicted up to 200 million world-wide deaths from 'bird flu' (H5N1) but there were only 74 deaths, all in SE Asia.

---

1   [https://www.nature.com/articles/d41586-020-01685-y]

With training and experience in clinical medicine and medical research, we (the authors) in contrast look for a medical solution to the problem with emphasis on improving resistance, the internal defensive immunity of all individuals, including the vulnerable. The government and its advisors have failed to mention enhancing our natural immunity, just by-passing it by the use of vaccines. It is necessary to understand immunity.

Ethnicity and Covid-19

Indonesia lies in the tropics, and has a population that is 90% Muslim. Yet publications from the Covid-19 pandemic have revealed that in Indonesia only 49.7% of a sample who were ill from this virus had a blood 25(OH)D level above 30ng/ml (75nmol/L). [Ref 15] The situation was even worse in the Philippines, also in the tropics, where only 26.2% of a sample who were ill had a blood Vitamin D level above 30ng/ml. [Ref 16] In India only 19.3% of a sample who were ill had blood Vitamin D level above 30ng/ml. [Ref 17]. This is a serious problem in these countries, but the problem becomes even greater when residents move to north-west Europe, as many of them do.

There are great ethnic variations in the incidence rate of Covid-19 and also in the death rates. But incidence and death rates do not always match: for example, in Russia on May 26th there had been 362,342 cases, an incidence rate of 2487 per million population. The UK had experienced 265,227 cases, 3929 per million. In Russia the corresponding deaths were 3807 (26 per million population) and in the UK 37,048 deaths (549 per million). This 30-fold disparity in death rates is a mystery, which may have more to do with politics than medicine.

Ethnicity and deaths; professional reluctance to face the obvious

The most striking observation in the UK is that the death rate from Covid-19 infection is much higher in the BAME (black, Asian, minority ethnicity) members of the population. *'More than 16% of coronavirus victims in England from BAME communities'* ran the headline in the London Evening Standard on April 20th. *'British BAME Covid-19 death rate more than twice that of whites'*, in The Guardian on May 1st. There were many similar newspaper headlines, but the UK Government has refused to comment.

The UK Office of National Statistics (ONS) produced its data May 7th. [Ref 18] The impression was confirmed, with ethnic black and Bangladeshi people showing a particularly high case mortality of more than four times the white population. The UK ONS used census data linkage to identify ethnicity of those who had died as it is not recorded on death certificates. The same thing has been observed in the USA, with a high risk of death among African Americans. This has likewise been downplayed, with efforts made to stop recording ethnicity in death reports.

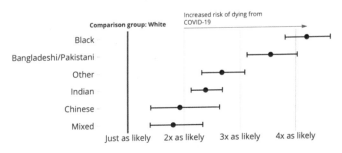

Ethnic risk of death from Covid-19 – UK Males ONS

Then we read; '*Among the first 15 deaths due to Covid-19 in Stockholm County, Sweden, six were reported by the Swedish-Somali Medical Society to be of Somali origin. Considering that only 0.84% of the Stockholm County population was born in Somalia this is an astonishingly high rate.*' The report (highlighted in the British Medical Journal on March 19th) discussed socio-economic factors, but not exclusively. It continued: '*In order to cope with the Covid-19 epidemic, preventive measures could be administration of vitamin D to high-risk populations, e.g. dark-skinned adults with low sun-exposure and/or individuals with risk factors for respiratory tract infections. Although it may not always be helpful, it is unlikely to be harmful.*' [Ref 19]

An explanation of the high number deaths in BAME people was called for and a number of pundits commented in the media. The answer was always sociological: socio-economic disadvantage, overcrowded houses, low-paid jobs, racism – all things that could not possible be corrected within the timescale of the pandemic. Biology was not mentioned, but regrettably scientific understanding in the UK is abysmally low, especially in Parliament. Meanwhile more people were dying, so immediate action was needed. Birmingham hospitals and the Labour Party set up independent inquiries, a process bound to take longer than the pandemic would last. Yet there was a serious paradox that effectively invalidated the provisional socio-economic explanation.

Medical deaths in the UK and the importance of the anomaly

As Thomas Kuhn pointed out, a paradox, an anomaly, is vital for the progression of science: '*Discovery commences with the awareness of anomaly.'* [Ref 20] We think of the world in a series of hypotheses, which represent the best way in which we can understand it. And so when we observe that 16% of deaths form Covid-19 are BAME, and we know much of the relative socio-economic disadvantage, we will assume that this is the cause of the excess deaths. But then we come across the uncomfortable anomaly.

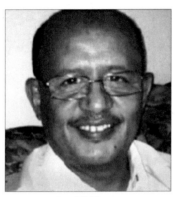

Dr El Tayar
Died March 25th 2020

In the UK over March, April, and May at least 26 doctors who contracted Covid-19 died, the first being the organ transplant surgeon Dr El Tayar on March 25th. [Ref 21] [Appendix 3] It is remarkable, and surely not a coincidence, that 25 of these doctors were BAME. The vital anomaly (which even ethnic commentators have carefully ignored) is that they are far from poor, or socially disadvantaged, and doctors are unlikely to live in overcrowded homes. What is the reason for this phenomenon?

The most obvious explanation is deficiency of Vitamin D, but this has not been mentioned in the media, by Government, or even in the medical journals. The ONS looked at linked records and concluded that the overall BAME excess mortality is not due to pre-existent diabetes or heart disease, and suggested a genetic predisposition. Yet we are not dealing with a homogenous group, but with people from diverse ethnic ancestry. Of the doctors who died, some were of African ethnicity, some of Indian, some Pakistani, some from the Middle East, and others from South-east Asia. Yes, there is something genetic that they have in common despite wide geocultural origins: it is genetically determined darker skin.

Professionals in denial

It is as though society (including Medicine) is frightened to say this. We know (or should know) that Vitamin D levels are lower in BAME people; that this is a risk factor for some infections; that Vitamin D has a vital role in defensive immunity, and its essential escalation during a serious infection. But the 'official' medical community has remained silent. As a result people have not received the Vitamin D supplement that has a strong foundation, is safe, cheap, and could be made available immediately. BAME people continue to die, yet strangely the deaths of BAME doctors have stopped abruptly. Conversations that DG has had with several ethnic Asian doctors in Blackburn (where his Vitamin D advice has been reported in the local newspaper, the Lancashire Telegraph) [Ref 22] indicate that such doctors are now taking Vitamin D supplements, and giving the same advice to their patients, despite official silence. The advice given by DG in this way appears to have cascaded locally with benefit to the local community. ONS has reported deaths by local authority in the UK: it records Covid-19 deaths per 100,000 in Blackburn-with-Darwen 29, lower than in neighbouring industrial towns with a large ethnic Asian community, such as Preston 34, Bolton 45, Bury 48, Chorley 37. Salford recorded a very high death rate at 98 per 100,000. Ribble Valley, where DG lives, has a very low Covid-19 death rate of just 11 per 100,000. It is a farming area centred on the market town of Clitheroe,

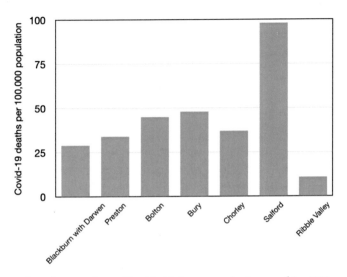

Death rates from Covid-19 in towns in Lancashire UK

with very little industry and a very small ethnic Asian community. [Ref 23]

In mid-April, one of us (DA), contacted Professor Parag Singhal, Professor of Endocrinology at Weston Super Mare and Hon Secretary of an 7,000-member organisation called the British Association of Doctors of Indian Origin (BAPIO). Both of us agreed that the BAME death rate, and unwillingness to confront it in the Press or by the Government was appalling, to the point of negligence. As already mentioned doses of 100,000units of Vitamin D3, in 1 ml vials for oral or intramuscular use are available in pharmacies over the counter in Italy, and we had already given some to hospital staff in the local Covid-19 hospital, so we decided to offer these to BAPIO doctors, and to date a total of 600 vials have been dispatched for distribution by BAPIO. The response has been very positive, and there have been no complaints of any side effects. And we continue to work with Parag who clearly thinks like we do.

Covid-19 and Vitamin D

Vitamin D and the Covid-19 pandemic

It is obvious to sensible people that before the pandemic of Covid-19, Vitamin D was not tested specifically as a prevention of or treatment for it. Even in Medicine the retro-spectoscope isn't that powerful, yet that is what many medical commentators seem to expect before sanctioning the use of Vitamin D. However evidence of benefit is now available in the form of preliminary communications. These have come the far East, because this is where the pandemic started and so experience from there has been able to travel westwards even more quickly than the virus has spread.

Early warnings from the East

The first report of a role of Vitamin D in the outcome of Covid-19 was from the Philippines and came to our attention on March 28th. [Ref 16] It was reported by Dr. Mark Alippio, a clinical professor and medical radiation scientist in the College of Allied Health Sciences, Davao Doctors College. It looked at the outcome of 212 patients with Covid-19 in three South-east Asian hospitals. They had their blood levels of Vitamin D (ie 25(OH)D3 and D2 combined) tested: in 25.9% it was greater than 30ng/ml, in 37.7% between 20 and 30 and in 36.3% less than 20ng/ml. Almost three quarters were therefore Vitamin D deficient. Of those with blood levels of Vitamin D greater

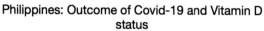

Philippines: Outcome of Covid-19 and Vitamin D status

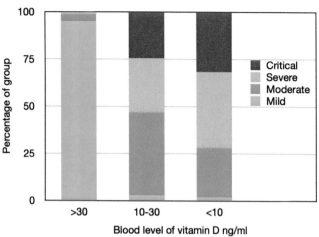

than 30ng/ml, 95% had just mild disease. Of those with lower blood levels of Vitamin D, only 3.6% had mild disease and the great majority had moderate, severe or critical disease. Vitamin D tests were not performed on those who had died. A blood level of Vitamin D greater than 30ng/ml was clearly a great advantage when facing Covid-19.

This early message should have given great encouragement to those in other countries responsible for treating patients with Covid-19. That was the purpose of this early communication, to inform physicians and governments in the West of what was happening in the East. We have no way of knowing if it influenced hospital practice in Europe, but it certainly did not influence UK Government policy. It has not been mentioned at any time by our Chief Medical Officer Professor Chris Whitty or our Chief Scientific Officer Professor Sir Patrick Vallance.

A second preliminary communication, from Indonesia, came to our attention on April 20th. [Ref 15] It studied 780 patients and investigated outcome, survival or death, based on Vitamin D status. Of 388 with blood levels of Vitamin D greater than 30ng/ml, 372 (96%) survived, and 16 (4%) died. Of the 213 with lower blood levels between 20 and 30ng/ml, 26 (12%) survived, and 187 (88%) died. Of the 179 with the lowest blood level of Vitamin D, less than 20ng/ml, only two (1%) survived and 177 (99%) died. This was indisputably important information sent to western nations that were struggling with the Covid-19 pandemic.

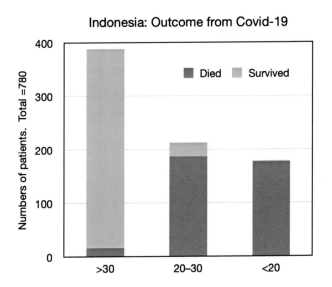

Indonesia: Outcome from Covid-19

Reaction from the UK and its paid advisers

By April 20th the UK had experienced 16,500 deaths from Covid-19. If we were to present the above information to the traditional man on the Clapham omnibus, and then ask if he would prefer to face Covid-19 with a blood level of Vitamin D of less than 10 or more than 30ng/ml, he would surely reply 'more than 30 please'. But the general public of the UK was not given a choice. There was official indifference, in fact negligent indifference. How many in the UK have had their blood levels of Vitamin D (25(OH) D, that is) checked, even on admission to hospital? There does seem to be more than a hint here of those in charge not just turning a blind eye, but of shutting two good ones.

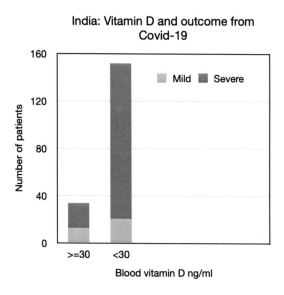

India: Vitamin D and outcome from Covid-19

A further brief study came from India. [Ref 17] Of 34 patients with blood Vitamin D levels equal to or greater than 30ng/ml, 13 (38%) had mild Covid-19 and 21 (62%) had a severe form. Of 142 with blood levels less than 30ng/ml, 21(15%) had mild disease and 121 (85%) had severe disease. We see the same pattern: it is of great benefit when ill with Covid-19 not to be deficient in Vitamin D.

The approach in the UK was, at least officially and in contrast to the Philippines, Indonesia and India, to avoid testing for Vitamin D, and not to intervene with other than supportive and intensive care in hospitals. It has been observed that obesity and diabetes indicate a bad outlook from Covid-19. [Ref 24] Unfortunately, it is not possible to influence these risk factors, both of which are known to be closely linked to Vitamin D deficiency. [Ref 25] Ethnicity has not been mentioned officially as a risk factor for death. Vitamin D deficiency has not been considered, even though information sent from the East identified this as the main and importantly, an immediately reversible risk factor.

Care for those in Care Homes

Age is a major risk factor for death from Covid-19, but is obviously not reversible. There have been 8.4 deaths per 100,000 aged under 65 years, compared to 286 deaths per 100,000 older than 65, meaning that pensioners are 34 times more likely to die from Covid-19. It is clear that a particular major risk factor for death is being old and especially if a resident in a care home. Such people are known to be deficient in Vitamin D. [Ref 26] How many of these residents (who never go outside) were given a supplement before or even when the pandemic reached the UK? In contrast, in Edmonton, Alberta an enlightened Dr Gerry Schwalfenberg looked after the residents of a care home. He had given them all a Vitamin D supplement of 2,000 units daily and subsequently checked their blood levels. A few were sub-optimal and so he gave a higher dose supplement. When the Covid-19 pandemic reached Edmonton he was able to report that none of his residents became ill from the virus, but this was not the experience in other care homes in the city. [Ref 27]

Such enlightened pragmatism has been absent in the UK, despite the Care Quality Commission (CQC) having jurisdiction over all care homes in the UK.

Need for universal Vitamin D supplementation

We have seen the extent of Vitamin D deficiency not just in the north-west of England, where we can blame the climate, but in also in tropical countries, where sun avoidance is the problem. Religious rules often demand extensive skin covering and it is unlikely that these rules will be changed. Vitamin D deficiency is considered to be the greatest global pandemic, affecting perhaps one billion people. It can be corrected.

We have seen that evolution indicates an ideal blood Vitamin D level of 40ng/ml (100nmol/ml) and we are fortunate in that we can now measure levels in all hospitals in the UK, as in many other countries. We emphasise again that an individual with a blood level of 10ng/ml might not appear to be at obvious immediate disadvantage. Yes, bone disease might be avoided, but there is no reserve for when a serious infection occurs. The Vitamin D requirement for steady-state bone health is much less than that required for escalation of immune defence mechanisms in response to serious infection; and we have already argued that calcium homeostasis will always dominate.

What is really required is enlightenment, by medical practitioners, religious leaders, and by governments with their public health advisors. There are priority groups who are likely to have Vitamin D deficiency. These are the elderly residents of care homes, those of BAME communities, the obese, those with diabetes, those whose religion demands covering of the skin. All people are at risk and those deficient in Vitamin D can be identified by a blood test, with the adequacy of the supplement checked by a repeat blood test.

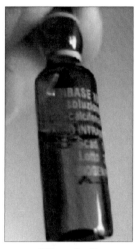

Vitamin D
100,000 units

A supplement of 2,000 to 4,000 units per day will usually achieve the target level. Alternatives are 20,000 units once week, or 100,000 units once a month. For people who would not accept a gelatine capsule, the 100,000 dose is an oil in a vial, and the oil can be taken either by mouth or as an injection. Vitamin D 100,000 units in 1ml in a single dose is the safe way to become replete in Vitamin D immediately for two months.

Response to the need for Vitamin D

Government, medical groups (such as the Royal Colleges of Physicians and the Society for Endocrinology), and most ethnic groups have shown a complete lack of enthusiasm for protecting the public against Covid-19 by enhancing natural immunity in this obvious way.

The UK Government and the NHS gets advice on Vitamin D from the Scientific Advisory Committee on Nutrition (SACN). In 2016 the Vitamin D Subcommittee produced a 289-page report that gave a good summary of Vitamin D, but identified its main purpose as being bone health and it did not discuss in any detail the role in immune-modulation.

The problem is once again that we can easily examine the (dominant) biochemistry of bone metabolism but not that of immunity. As a general rule, we measure what is easiest not what is most important. Yet we should accept what basic science of cytogenetics tells us about the importance of Vitamin D. We must recognise its blood levels as nature and evolution determined, and as the studies in the Philippines, Indonesia, and India have informed us during the Covid-19 pandemic. We must hope that further research is being performed now in Europe and other continents. The Covid-19 pandemic has given a remarkable opportunity for research into the role of Vitamin D in immunity, and we hope this is not being lost.

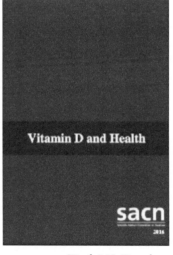

Fortunately, despite the lack of advice from official bodies, there are signs of growing grass-roots awareness, as many are making their own choice. They are reading occasional reports in the newspapers. [Ref 22] Do they want to risk serious or even fatal Covid-19, or do they choose to take a Vitamin D supplement that might reduce this risk? On the advice given, there is no risk from Vitamin D, cost about just £1 per month. Not a bad investment if it saves your life.

The Concept of proof

We have heard and read countless negative statements about Vitamin D, by people who seem totally ignorant of its evolution and cytogenetics, are unaware of its role in immune defence, and who see it as uniquely about bone health and the avoidance of rickets.

They usually say 'There is no proof that Vitamin D is of benefit in Covid-19'. Of course not. With a virus that is new to humankind, how could major studies have been undertaken? These mechanisms are precisely to defend us from unknown viruses. When they see the provisional reports from the Philippines, Indonesia, and India, they say, (as in BBC Radio 4 '*More or Less*' on Wednesday May 13th), that the reports are 'only' provisional, and that 'they have not yet been peer-reviewed'. An observant Hong Kong schoolgirl cleared a whole beach in Phuket in 2004 Boxing Day tsunami, when the sea suddenly went out, because she had heard about tsunamis in class at school. Would you accept such a schoolgirl's tsunami warning by moving to higher ground, or would you wait on the beach for peer review, and be drowned while waiting? Here we are in the midst of a pandemic with more than 40,000 deaths from Covid-19 in the UK alone, and those paid to live in Ivory Towers seem to be blissfully unaware of the real world.

The demand for a randomised controlled trial (RCT) of any treatment for Covid-19, was stated by senior member of the WHO Ivory Tower on BBC television on Sunday morning May 17th, without so much as mentioning Vitamin D. To demand one for Vitamin D is unrealistic. It would take about a year to design and to find funding for such an RCT. Recruitment would follow, but this must be with informed consent. In respect of Covid-19, would a volunteer accept that present evidence shows a very important benefit from a good blood level of Vitamin D, but a high risk of death from a low level? Who would be happy to be allocated to the placebo? Or would informed consent be withheld?

An RCT from many centres in the USA was reported in 2019, before the Covid-19 pandemic and thus of limited value at the present time. It has however been presented to us by the Royal College of Physicians of London as 'evidence' that Vitamin D would not be of value in Covid-19 infection, thus justifying its silent inaction. In this study 1360 critically ill patients with high risk of death, who had been tested to be Vitamin D deficient, were randomised so that half received Vitamin D 540,000 units as a single enteral dose. Analysis showed no benefit. [Ref 28] The paper made no mention of the underlying diseases that caused these patients to be critically ill and they obviously formed a heterogenous group. The paper was curiously titled 'Early High-Dose Vitamin D_3 for Critically ill, Vitamin D-Deficient Patients'. If a person is critically ill the underlying disease is obviously very advanced, and in the title the first word 'Early' (which carries the greatest impact) should be replaced by 'Late', something that should have been noted by those peers of the prestigious New England Journal of Medicine who did the reviewing. This paper does not negate our contention that in face of the pandemic of Covid-19 the government through its public health agencies should have given all citizens, and especially those at risk, Vitamin D in the most convenient and effective dose of 100,000 units, so as to prepare them for probable infection. It is our 'Mission Statement' to prevent Covid-19 infection from escalating from asymptomatic or mild disease into critical or fatal disease. We are not proposing to prevent infection itself, but to reduce serious illness and death. We are also not proposing to rescue critically ill patients from the jaws of death, but we wish that we could. The above-mentioned paper proves nothing concerning Vitamin D and Covid-19 infection.

Few seem to be aware of the meaning of proof. It comes from the Ancient Greek mathematician Euclid, and it means the fulfilment of pre-determined criteria. So we must throw back the question and ask: 'What criteria of proof would you accept?' A rigorous concept of proof was used by Robert Koch in his recognition of the microbial cause of tuberculosis, but he found that it lacked sensitivity. He was unable to 'prove' that cholera was due to a micro-organism, although it was accepted at the time on the basis of less rigorous and less formal criteria.

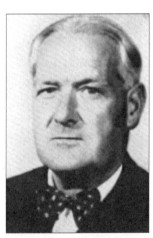

Sir Austin Bradford Hill

Proof is pragmatic, and there is more to it than the hallowed RCT. Proof is rarely absolute: acceptance of, for example, the proposition that Vitamin D enhances immunity and helps protect against serious infection, relies on judgement. This has been expanded by Sir Austin Bradford Hill, who developed series of criteria that are very important in making a judgement [Ref 29]. Consider the proposal that cigarette smoking causes lung cancer [Ref 30]: no-one doubts this, but how strong is the evidence? Has it been proven? The 'weight of evidence' certainly leads to an acceptance that cigarette smoking causes lung cancer. Is the proposal that Vitamin D enhances immunity and helps protect against serious infection weaker or stronger?

The importance of Pragmatic Judgement

In his investigation with Sir Richard Doll that lung cancer might be caused by cigarette smoking, Bradford Hill recognised that it is not always possible to conduct clinical experiments, randomised controlled clinical trials. Nevertheless he felt that it is necessary to make decisions and not to dither with self-righteous

> **Bradford Hill's Criteria**
>
> Strength of association
>
> Consistency of association
>
> Temporality
>
> Biological gradient
>
> Plausibility
>
> Coherence
>
> Experimentation
>
> Analogy

inaction, and it was to help with decision-making that he produced his criteria. We feel that our contention that Vitamin D is of value in preventing Covid-19 from progressing from an asymptomatic or mild illness to serious or fatal illness fulfils the Criteria. Judgement means acting on the basis on incomplete information: it is our judgement that Vitamin D is of value in preventing serious or fatal Covid-19, and therefore we (the authors) take a regular supplement and we advise our families and friends to do the same. With the knowledge that we have accumulated, and that we have tried to pass on in this book, would anyone decline to take Vitamin D? Are Boris Johnson and his infected advisers shunning, or covertly

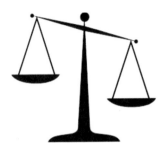

using Vitamin D? It would be revealing to know; after all one of us (DA) did write to tell him.

Courts of Law are accustomed to making a decision without 'conclusive' proof. They make a judgement on the basis of probability, a decision of 'beyond reasonable doubt'. It is our assessment that the weight of evidence is in favour of the proposal that Vitamin D enhances immunity and is very likely to protect against serious or fatal Covid-19. Those against the proposal appear to be ignorant of the facts or they simply say 'I don't think so', or 'I do not find the (unread) evidence compelling'.

Response to the Coronavirus pandemic

Retrospect on how the pandemic was handled

The strange thing is how the Government through its medical and scientific advisors is apparently ignorant of the role of Vitamin D in escalating the defensive immune response to serious infection. Even after more than two months of what we hope would have included intellectual activity, there has been no official consideration of its potential value. Other official bodies such as the medical Royal Colleges refuse even to debate the issue. Why is this? Why should the proposal to use the cheap and readily-available Vitamin D be ignored in such a comprehensive way? Is this a conspiracy? Is it because it is too cheap, or too simple an answer? Is it because it would have made unnecessary expensive projects for testing antiviral agents and vaccines, which are under the control of big pharmaceutical companies, and receive lucrative funding from governments?

Conspiracy of Silence?

Or is the conspiracy of silence even more sinister? The deaths of certain groups, for example the 25 BAME out of 26 doctors who died from Covid-19 could be regarded as negligence by the UK Government, its advisors, and its public health bodies. They must have known about the functions of Vitamin D in immunity and its serious deficiency in BAME groups in particular. Unless they were asleep they must have been aware of preliminary information coming from the Philippines, Indonesia, and India. It was surely serious negligence to fail to act on this knowledge in the face of rapidly escalating death rates serious enough to close down a large part of the national economy. Therefore, the Government and its advisors must be very concerned about a threat of legal claims of negligence, with a massive financial impact and that seriously undermines their credibility. The simplest way to prevent this is to pretend that Vitamin D does not exist.

There is no doubt that some aspects of the pandemic were handled badly and uncritically. The outcome would have been very different had Vitamin D been used. The lockdown would have made some sense had it been combined with a concerted and specific effort to measure and correct widespread Vitamin D-deficiency, at least in those most at risk of exposure to coronavirus.

Death of a transplant surgeon

Although the excess of deaths and serious Covid-19 became obvious early in the UK experience, the first doctor to die from Covid-19 was Dr El Tayar, a 63 year-old transplant surgeon in London. [Ref 21] He died on March 25th and his death was reported in the press on the following day. More were to follow, but there was no response from the government or the medical bodies to examine this serious anomaly. [Appendix 3]

To set up a committee of investigation is the natural response of Government, if only to give the illusion that something is being done. The urgency of the situation was ignored, despite the fact that 500 UK citizens were dying each day. The investigation could have taken place, but in the meantime a potential benefit of Vitamin D could have

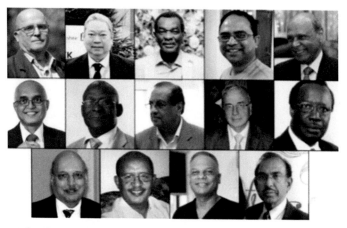

The first BAME doctors to die from Covid-19 in the UK

been broadcast. After all, details of DNA antigen tests, antibody tests, hydroxychloroquine, anti-virals, various vaccines had all been publicised, but not the natural substance Vitamin D.

The UK national public health bodies decided to recommend Vitamin D in a minimal dose 400units per day 'to compensate for remaining indoors during lockdown, so as to help keep bones, teeth and muscles healthy'. Not a mention of immunity. [Ref 31] To recommend ten times this dose (perfectly safe according to SACN) might have been expected to become a government responsibility. This would have taken a long time to set up, with supplies to be sought and distribution to be organised. However with the annual cost of 4,000 units per day being only about £10, and its readily availability on the internet, with adequate publicity its rapid acquisition could have been left to individuals. This would have been taken up more by the young and the 'middle classes', and so a public health initiative would have been necessary to make certain that it was available to the whole population. And especially to those at greatest risk, the elderly in residential care, for whom provision of Vitamin D should have taken priority. It could have been done through the Care Quality Commission, but was not. The nation initially ignored and then just watched as the frail elderly people died. We accept that their natural deaths were not too distant, but Vitamin D would have offered them (and their families), and support staff, better protection than just locking them away in isolation.

Lockdown

Government policy during the pandemic in the UK and other countries was determined by mathematicians, who naturally used numbers to dictate what to do. We could hardly expect them to know about the cytogenetics of Vitamin D in the escalation of defensive immunity. Lockdown involved not just locking the doors of residential care homes, but keeping us all in our houses, stopping work for most people, closing universities, schools, churches, mosques, synagogues, and stopping sporting activities and airline travel. Lockdown did not affect the employment of those who designed it. The cost has been enormous, but has it been successful?

Lockdown was introduced in the UK on March 23rd 2020, when there had been an 'alarming' 284 deaths from Covid-19. Six weeks later the number had risen to 30,000, an increase by a factor of more than 100. We are told that without lockdown the number of deaths would have been even greater, but given the experience of other countries this is unlikely. One of us (DG) has a friend who is a devout Christian. She prays to God every day that the

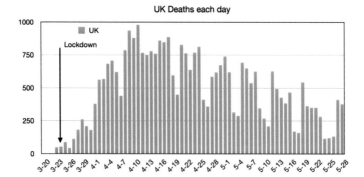

UK Deaths each day

pandemic will come to an end, as would have happened in ancient times, but she draws the line at human sacrifice. When questioned about the effectiveness of her prayers she says that without them the pandemic would have been much worse. Which works best, lockdown or prayer? Or are they both ineffective?

It is not in the nature of government or any official body to admit to error. It was perhaps reasonable to introduce lockdown on March 23rd, but it should be admitted that it has not been successful. Reflective practice should be the norm. After all, there is an alternative way to protect the public and restart the economy: Vitamin D. Lockdown should have been accompanied by an immediate Vitamin D policy.

Is it that only a vaccine pays?

There seems to be a conspiracy of silence, with no discussion by government, medical profession or press, of the potential role of Vitamin D to help solve the Covid-19 pandemic. It is as if the solution must be difficult, but as with the Manhattan Project, governments believe there is nothing that money cannot solve. Thus, the D-book stays closed. This is good for academics, who need funds in order to survive. We see that the funding in the UK goes to such august places as Imperial College London and the University of Oxford, institutions for whom humble Vitamin D may be too simple and cheap. The simplest way to make Vitamin D go away is to pretend it was never there anyway. But does coronavirus agree with this analysis?

Extracts from a letter from DA to Bill Gates, April 9th 2020....

'I know you are an independent thinker and.... likely to listen to common sense.... Coronavirus is exploiting a widespread and easily rectified defect in our capacity to mount a defensive immune response. Alas, our medical and public health institutions have failed to recognise the risks of widespread Vitamin D deficiency.... Vitamin D3, the animal version, can only be formed by ultraviolet irradiation of 7-dehydrocholesterol on the skin. This *cleaves... the B ring, the molecule opens up, and isomerises to D3 (cholecalciferol) in which form it travels to the liver for conversion into 25(OH)D3, the storage form.... Evolutionally, 1,25(OH)2D3 is vital for calcium transport, even in unicellular organisms.... In mammals, the best appreciated is its role as a hormone that... takes priority over all local functions... With adequate levels of 25(OH) D3, a normal immune system can mount an effective response against viruses of all kinds, including the coronavirus. But at this time of year, and for many reasons, Vitamin D deficiency is rife. Thus, it should be no surprise to read that in Chicago and New Orleans, where 30% of the population is black, this subgroup accounts for 70% of the deaths. Dark-skinned individuals are especially prone to Vitamin D deficiency because their melanin acts as a natural sunblock.... We will only overcome this global catastrophe if we address the question of Vitamin D deficiency on a global scale, and with great urgency, and so convert Coronavirus from the killer it is in the Vitamin D-deficient, back to the tame upper respiratory tract virus, which in most people with adequate D3 levels just causes a bad cold.*

'...Your Foundation could help enormously by facilitating...use of sensible doses of Vitamin D3, such as I suggest in my film (https://youtu.be/ ga0QCAu_bic). For your information, in Italy Vitamin D3 100,000units in olive oil is licensed for over the counter purchase,.. and marketed under the trade name DIBASE. In the UK the regulatory authorities, fearing overdosing (which requires a hundred times more) make sensible doses

of Vitamin D3 only available with great difficulty on prescription! ...It would cost a mere 40 million Euros to render immediately the whole of Italy Vitamin D-sufficient for 3 months! And it needs no controlled trials first. I do hope you will take this seriously, and treat it with the urgency that is called for, but is singularly lacking globally.'

There was no reply from Bill Gates, who is of course, very busy organising vaccines.

Some pertinent observations from Vanessa Beeley

We owe a great deal to this journalist for her two recent articles in *OffGuardian*. [Ref 32] Here is a pertinent excerpt:

'The newly emerging statistics are now increasingly... pointing to the futility and negative consequences of lockdown.... It is now accepted that there is a high mortality rate among the elderly in Care Homes in the UK and globally among the same elderly civilians who are being 'asked' to sign DNRs (Do Not Resuscitate forms). That amounts to signing their own death warrant, should they present any of the Covid–19 symptoms. They will be neglected, isolated from their families when at their most vulnerable and left alone to die, even though it is possible that they have not contracted the virus...'

Beeley identifies that government policy appears to have been formulated by Professor Neil Ferguson, who entered our story earlier. His mathematical model was accepted and recommended by the WHO for international use. Ferguson is acting director of the Vaccine Impact

Modelling Consortium (VIMC), which is based at Imperial College in London.

Vaccine development

Government policy is overwhelmingly directed towards the development of a vaccine, in co-operation with variety of multinational organisations. But there is something about vaccines that the reader should understand. A vaccine is directed against a specific micro-organism which itself must be known. Vaccines are very useful against endemic infections, that is to say infections that are continually within society. These include measles, mumps, rubella, pertussis, human papilloma virus (HPV), hepatitis B virus (HBV), typhoid, polio (on the verge of eradication), and smallpox (now eradicated).

But this is not possible against extraneous infections that cause epidemics. It would have been impossible to have protected the world against Covid-19 by developing a vaccine, as the virus was unknown until December 2019. It inevitably takes many months and so by the time the vaccine is available the pandemic will be at an end.

There is also the challenge of testing such a new vaccine, which is not just about efficacy. Safety is also of paramount importance as it is imperative to do no harm, although a very rare side-effect affecting one in a million cannot be avoided. But a large number of people must receive a vaccine for a side-effect of one in a thousand to be recognised, and such effects may not be immediate. We should be wary of the experience of Pandemrix, a vaccine that was introduced at the time of Swine Flu in 2009/10. It was developed hastily but received a licence from the European Medicines Agency. It was given to six million people in Europe, without a randomised controlled trial.

After some delay, it was considered by the UK Health & Safety Executive (now Public Health England, PHE) to be the cause of what has been described as a minor epidemic of narcolepsy, a brain disorder characterised by attacks of uncontrollable deep sleep. The licence was withdrawn in 2014. Great care is therefore needed in the future.

When the pandemic has passed, how can we test a vaccine for effectiveness? Would it be on the basis of a randomised controlled trial (RCT) with informed consent, given the demand for this in respect of Vitamin D? This would inevitably create an additional administration burden and a long delay. The disease incidence might then be so low that there would too few cases to draw a statistically valid conclusion. If in the interests of expediency a vaccine were to administered without an RCT, and if the pandemic were not to return, would we attribute this to the vaccine? Remember that the previous pandemics of Spanish Flu, Asian Flu, and Hong Kong Flu went away without return and without vaccines.

Vitamin D and Vaccines compared

Vaccines therefore appear to us not to be appropriate for pandemics. What is required is to protect the population immediately against any and all previously unknown viruses. Vitamin D, through mechanisms described above, is nature's tried and tested way to escalate our front-line immune defensive response to all micro-organisms. The only rational and scientifically honest approach to the present and future pandemics is therefore to offer Vitamin D to the whole population in a dose sufficient to achieve ideal and tested blood levels, so as to protect against new infections from the outset. Therefore, it is essential to confront almost universal Vitamin D deficiency.

A direct approach to the UK government's relevant advisers

In a direct approach to the chief medical and scientific advisors, on March 29th 2020 DA wrote to Professor Chris Whitty and Sir Patrick Vallance, *'These four papers [Refs 6,11,12,13] are accessible on the internet and together show the importance of Vitamin D in the immune response to infection, and the safety of a single dose of 100,000 Units of Vitamin D3 orally to restore 25(OH)D3 to levels needed by the immune system. This is a simple measure to help fight a desperate situation, and it will cost very little and may save thousands of lives'*. No reply was received.

We will see that there is a huge international effort to produce vaccines. Of course, the primary intention is to help humankind, but there is also much money to be made by participants, and therefore additional extraneous motivation, and so conflicts of interest. The system involves networks of organisations, governments, alliances, and mechanisms of funding.

VIMC and GAVI

VIMC (Vaccine Impact Modelling Consortium) is hosted by Bill and Melinda Gates, as is GAVI (Global Alliance for Vaccines and Immunisation). The Gates Foundation also launched the Global Health Leaders Launch Decade of Vaccines Collaboration (GHLLDVC). By the end of 2018 Imperial College (where VIMC is based) had received $185 million from the Gates Foundation.

GAVI receives additional funds from the World Bank, with donor Governments, of which the UK is the largest, pledging £1.44 billion for 2016-2020. During the first week in June 2020, Boris Johnson, on behalf of the UK Government, hosted a virtual conference from London. The Global Vaccination Market revenue is projected (before Covid) to reach $59.2 billion this year. *'Vaccines are set to be a major source of income for the world's largest pharmaceutical corporations, and the British Government has invested in that lucrative future'*, writes Vanessa Beeley. [Ref 23]

CEPI

CEPI (Coalition for Epidemic Preparedness Innovations) was launched in Davos in 2017 by the governments of Norway and India, the Bill & Melinda Gates Foundation, the Wellcome Trust global health charity, and the World Economic Forum. It has received funding from the governments of Germany, Japan, Australia, the UK, Belgium, and Canada.

Our Chief Medical Officer Professor Chris Whitty, (who is also a Consultant Physician at University College, London), chairs the UK Vaccine Network, and co-leads for the National Institute for Health Research, which has given another £20 million to CEPI for Covid-19 Vaccine development. Such a sum in March 2020 would have gone a long way to protect the UK population against the most damaging effects of the Covid-19 pandemic. Those who suffered most were those who due to Vitamin D deficiency had the weakest Vitamin D-dependent antiviral systems.

The WHO tells us *'Be sure to consult trusted and credible sources, like your health worker, local health authorities, health institutions like NHS.UK, Public Health England, WHO or the members of the Vaccine*

Safety Net'. (It might have added *'And at all costs steer clear of time-expired has-beens like the dangerous Davids, Anderson and Grimes!'*)

We may therefore well ask how much is the UK Government's policy to lockdown guided by genuine medical expert opinion and how much by commercial, Big Pharma, interests and agendas? Members of SAGE (the Scientific Advisory Group for Emergencies) were described as *'shocked, concerned and worried for the impartiality of advice'* after the Prime Minister's Chief Adviser Dominic Cummings effectively gatecrashed their meetings. The fact that Cummings used his influence to politicise the SAGE meetings should alert us to the possibility of political exploitation of Covid–19.

Ignorance or ignoring

Unexpected attitudes

We have presented information about the immune-modulating function of Vitamin D, and also some important early-warning information concerning the outcome of Covid-19 in relationship to body stores of Vitamin D, measured by blood levels of 25(OH)D. We are not alone, and there are groups of doctors in the UK and the USA with like concerns, but when it comes to official spokesmen there is a deafening silence.

Why is this? Why do senior doctors and scientists seem to be completely ignorant of and disinterested in the issues that we have highlighted? Is such ignorance wide-spread in medical science? Has something gone seriously wrong with medical education and current medical practice? Has curiosity been completely suppressed? Why do we have apathy in the face of a serious epidemic? Or are we, the authors, living through a bad dream of a pandemic of Covid-19? Might it be that one day we will wake up, rub our eyes, and see that all is well after all? Might we be mistaken?

We have attempted to engage in debate with medical journals, with government advisors, with politicians, with national newspapers but with no response. We have tried to stimulate interest by the Royal Colleges of Physicians of London (RCP) and Edinburgh. After several attempts and rejections, we were able to receive an agreement for our letter (written also with Professor Parag Singhal) to be published in the college journal 'College Commentary'. Our main concern has been mentioned. It is the Vitamin D report by SACN, published in 2016, which is concerned about the role of Vitamin D in bone health, but it is very fleeting in its discussion of it immune-modulating effects. It fails to mention the cytogenetics of Vitamin D that is vital in the escalation of defensive immunity. [Ref 34] It fails to acknowledge the need for reserves of 25(OH)D at the time of serious infection. Our letter was to criticise the SACN report as inadequate at the time of the Covid-19 pandemic and plead for a revision beyond the vision of 'nutrition'.

It was considered by the RCP that it would not be appropriate for our letter to be published unless it were accompanied by a contrasting view, in other words that enlightenment must by matched by darkness.

Our letter is as follows:

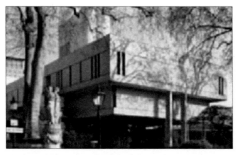

Royal College of Physicians of London

Critique of current SACN Guidelines on Vitamin D requirements (2016)

The Editor, College Commentary

Royal College of Physicians of London

Sir,

The above Guidelines [1] treat D3 mainly is as a vitamin, for which there is a partial dietary source, and whose main function is that of a hormone for musculoskeletal health. This diminishes the importance of its role in the immune system.

Back to first principles; evolution of Vitamin D3. [2]

Solar UVB radiation acts on 7-dehydrocholesterol, in the skin to form pre-D3, which immediately isomerises to cholecalciferol (Vitamin D3). This travels to the liver for 25-hydroxylation to the long-acting form, 25(OH)D3. The biologically active form 1,25(OH)2D3 is produced by 1-hydroxylation in the kidneys. Under the action of PTH it acts as a hormone for absorption and maintenance of blood ionised calcium. Its other essential roles include activation of cells of the immune system in the event of a viral infection, forming the vital first line of counter-attack.

Vitamin D3, and the healing of rickets

Vitamin D3 was discovered in the early 1900s through the healing power of sunshine on rickets and osteomalacia. The system of units was developed from rat bioassay, accounting for the dauntingly high numbers of noughts we find; 100,000 Units of D3 is in fact a mere 2.5 milligrams. In the 1960's further details of the 25- and 1-alpha hydroxylation steps of D3 in liver and kidneys respectively were worked out, and later the mechanism of action of 1,25(OH)2D3 via the vitamin D-receptor (VDR) on target tissues [2]. The 1,25(OH)2 D3–VDR heterodimer binds to sites on DNA, and leads to a cascade that promotes escalation of the immune response [3].

Production and action of Vitamin D3 in extra-endocrine tissues

1,25(OH)2D3 is also made by local intracellular 1-alpha hydroxylase, acting on 25(OH)D3 drawn from the general pool. Between October and March in the UK the sun's UVB rays are entirely filtered out by the atmosphere, and so we depend on reserves built up during the summer, when UVB light can penetrate down to ground level at midday [4]. To have adequate levels of circulating 25(OH)D3 by the late winter requires adequate solar exposure in the summer to raise 25(OH)D3 to around 100 ng/ml (250 nmol/l) by September. Even in light-skinned sunbathers this is unlikely to be achieved, and so it follows that everyone requires Vitamin D3 supplementation, at least during the winter.

Are 25(OH)D3 requirements of extra-endocrine systems the same?

PTH levels vary cyclically with the seasons, with highest levels in late winter, when 25(OH)D3 levels are lowest. The endocrine system will always have priority for 1,25(OH)2D3 that is produced by the kidneys from meagre levels of 25(OH)D3. Under virus attack the immune system will work best if there is a high normal level of 25(OH)D3 [5]. In times of deficiency of 25(OH)D3 the endocrine system will always dominate, to preserve a stable ionised calcium level in the blood. It is of paramount *importance for normal locomotion for the fight or flight reaction to have a stable circulating ionised calcium level.*

Implications for deciding the optimal levels of Vitamin D3 intake

It follows that the amount of D-supplement to produce an adequate blood level of 25(OH)D3 should be set higher for good immune function than the minimum needed to preserve bone health. It is extremely difficult to push Vitamin D3 intake or 25(OH)D3 too high [6], so we need to target the most susceptible, and not just the average population as is currently recommended. This is doubly important when we consider that our population is now more heterogeneous than ever, with regard to living conditions, summer solar exposure, ethnicity and skin pigmentation, and also to include a wide range of behavioural factors Including extreme clothing and sun block.

Evidence that Vitamin D3 deficiency influences severity of COVID-19.

First, there is substantial agreement that seasonal Vitamin D3-deficiency predisposes to upper and lower respiratory infections in general [7,8].

Second, it has become increasingly apparent during the current pandemic that those who dying are the most D-deficient. In Italy (where solar-avoidance is widespread) the pandemic started in the North, in the prosperous area of Bergamo, where there is serious air pollution. By late March reports in the popular press stated that those dying of Covid-19 were severely D-deficient. In the USA there is a disproportionate number of African Americans, an effect attributed to social deprivation. In the UK, there is a disproportionate death rate among ethnic Asians in London and elsewhere [9] and this also applies to doctors, who are not socially-deprived. Of the first 26 doctors to die no less than 25 were Black, Asian or Minority Ethnic (BAME). And now not a day goes by without another report, from different parts of the World with strong evidence to link a high mortality rate to a high D-deficiency rate. Clearly, in the D-replete, coronavirus mostly just gives a nasty cold-like illness. But with D-deficiency, it breaks through to wreak havoc in the lower respiratory tract, and kills [10].

How do the SACN Guidelines stand up to scrutiny?

In 2007 the Committee just considered the very young, the pregnant and lactating, and the very old, assuming that others would have adequate solar exposure. It concluded they should take 10 mcg daily (400 IU /d) of Vitamin D. In 2010 the SACN agreed to reconsider Dietary Reference Values because of advice to stay out of the sun and use sunblocks. In 2016 this advice was extended to all ages, still based solely on perceived musculoskeletal needs.

What, if anything, needs to be changed in the SACN guidelines?

Musculoskeletal and immune-enhancing functions of vitamin D require different considerations, but the SACN report of 2016 fails to do this. In fact, if the immune-enhancing functions of vitamin D are to receive the attention that they deserve, they *should surely be considered under a Scientific Advisory Committee for Immune Defence (SACID), something made clear by the number of deaths resulting from COVID-19. This would obviously provide better preparation for a second wave of this epidemic and for the inevitable epidemics in the future.*

Need for immediate action

We suggest that urgent approval be given to make available Vitamin D3 in orally doses of up to 100,000IU (2.5 mg). As a single dose this would safely restore 25(OH)D3 levels to normal for at least 2 months. This should most urgently be applied to health care workers and others exposed to coronavirus patients; to other individuals at high risk of Vitamin D3 deficiency; to residents of nursing homes; and to individuals suffering from or recovering from coronavirus infection.

References:
1 = [Ref 47], 2=[Ref 6], 3=[Ref 15], 4=[Ref 47], 5=[Ref 13], 6,7,8=[Ref 47], 9=[21], 10 https://www.thelancet.com/article/S1473-3099(20)30086-4/fulltext

The replies:

From Dr Adrienne Cullum, head of nutrition science at Public Health England (PHE)

'The existing vitamin D advice is focused on musculoskeletal health. The Scientific Advisory Committee on Nutrition (SACN) considered the evidence on Vitamin D and infection to be insufficient and highlighted that high intakes above 100 micrograms per day may be harmful.*

PHE and SACN are monitoring any emerging evidence on nutrition and COVID19 and assessing its quality. Limited UK evidence published to date on Covid19 and Vitamin D suggests there is no association. We reissued our advice on Vitamin D supplementation at the beginning of April 2020, which was published on NHS UK. As the stay at home restrictions are gradually eased, our advice remains that some groups, such as those in shielded groups and living in care homes, should continue to take a daily supplement containing 10 micrograms of Vitamin D.'

Background:

- *Current advice on Vitamin D is based on the recommendations of the Scientific Advisory Committee on Nutrition (SACN) following its review of the evidence on Vitamin D and health.*

- *In order to protect musculoskeletal health, SACN recommended that the blood concentration of all individuals in the UK should not fall below 25 nmol/L at any time of the year and gave advice on the Vitamin D intake required to support this.*

- *In its report on Vitamin D and Health, SACN concluded that evidence on Vitamin D and infection is inconsistent.*

- *Further references: SACN considered the evidence on Vitamin D and infection to be insufficient and highlighted that high intakes above 100 micrograms per day may be harmful (SACN, 2016) and example of UK evidence published to date on Covid19 and vitamin D (Hastie et al 2020).*

Joint statement on COVID-19 and vitamin D

'Since the onset of the pandemic, we have been contacted by some fellows of the RCP about vitamin D supplements. Due to the lack of exposure to sunlight caused by the lockdown and the possible role of vitamin D in immunity, some feel a national programme of high dose supplements, targeted at those at higher risk of vitamin D deficiency and COVID-19, would be appropriate.

'After a review of published data by our advisory group on nutrition, weight and health, the RCP, British Dietetic Association and the Society for Endocrinology have concluded that there is currently no evidence for recommending high doses for the general population. Further research should be undertaken as soon as possible to help us prepare advice in the event of a second wave of COVID-19.

'The RCP, British Dietetic Association and the Society for Endocrinology support the advice of Public Health England. As stated on the NHS website, everyone should consider taking 10 micrograms (400iu) of vitamin D a day to keep their bones and muscles healthy.

'This advice is particularly important for people from a BAME background. The higher the amount of melanin in the skin the less it absorbs UV radiation, which converts vitamin D into its active form.

'It is important to note that people with proven vitamin D deficiency, or specific medical conditions such as malabsorption or kidney failure may need higher doses or specific vitamin D preparations to ensure they have adequate levels of vitamin D.

'The NHS website also states that there is no evidence that vitamin D reduces the risk of developing COVID-19

*or modifying its clinical course. This is correct, and supported by **the recent rapid evidence review** by the Centre for Evidence Based Medicine at the University of Oxford and **Vitamin D and SARS-CoV-2 virus/ COVID-19 disease** by Lanham-New SA, Webb AR, Cashman KD, et al.*

'We support urgent research into any potential benefit that may be derived from vitamin D to prevent or help treat COVID-19 infection.'

On reflection

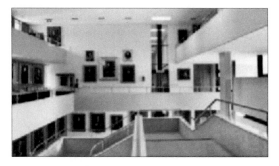

Royal College of Physicians of London

On reflection we view our letter (sent on May 8th 2020) to be based on fact and up-to-date biomedical science, and also reflecting the current pandemic of Covid-19 with in excess of 30,000 deaths with more reported each day. In contrast, the replies pay no attention to up-to-date biomedical science and are completely remote from the pandemic. We despair at the state of Medicine and the serious lack of leadership at the present time. We wonder what the readers of the journal will make of this 'balanced' exchange of letters. What is the balance of view? Is it in favour of the use of vitamin D in doses suggested to be

4,000 units daily or 100,000 units monthly, or on the other hand the SACN view of 400 units daily, with a higher dose above 100mcg (=4,000units) 'may be harmful'. This dose, which we recommend and is acknowledged to be safe, but what is meant by 'above 100mcg per day'? One hundred times that dose would be expected to cause problems. Our stated recommendation for immediate action was 100,000 units (2.5mg), sufficient for 'at least two months'.

The reply from Dr Adrienne Cullum of SACN mentions that the blood level of Vitamin D as 25(OH)D '...*should not fall below 25 nmol/L at any time of the year*'. This is a mere 10ng/ml, compared to the evolutionary ideal of 40ng/ml (100nmol/L). This is a dangerously low level, but if it is stated as a policy, it should be followed by advice that the population should be screened at regular intervals, especially people at high risk of vitamin D deficiency.

The 'Joint Statement' ends by '*We support urgent research into any potential benefit that may be derived from vitamin D to prevent or help treat COVID-19 infection*'. We, the authors of this book, support urgent action by the use of Vitamin D to enhance the immunity of the population who are at serious risk from Covid-19, but at the same time we would strongly support continuing research into the role of Vitamin D. There are currently great opportunities for research, and we hope these opportunities are being taken. Those who demand randomised controlled trials will need to move very quickly as the pandemic might well have come to an end before they are able to recruit (with informed consent) let alone reach a conclusion and have their paper peer-reviewed. There any many opportunities for careful observation of associations and temporality between Vitamin D with clinical and biochemical parameters of disease, and of course outcome.

We found the response to our letter to be dismal, unscientific, and irrelevant to the current pandemic. We feel that it can do nothing other than diminish the reputation of national medical organisations.

Is the response based on ignorance? If so it can be corrected by learning. Or is it based on ignoring? This is much more serious and cannot be corrected as it is part of personal or institutional weakness. Or could it be based on a hidden agenda? Is there something going on in the background that requires the denial of a role for Vitamin D in defensive immunity against infection? If so it must be coming from a high level.

The comment '*Limited UK evidence published to date...*' indicates an astounding degree of British arrogance. Yes, there is 'limited UK evidence' because research has not been and is not being undertaken in the UK. The vast majority of basic scientific and clinical research undertaken on Vitamin D in recent years has been outside the UK. To ignore this and the careful clinical observations in the Philippines, Indonesia, and India borders on the criminally negligent. Recent university league tables indicate the decline of academia in the UK and its rise in Asia.

Concluding thoughts

We are both retired and no longer registered with the General Medical Council, so any advice we give must be taken or rejected on its own merits and at the reader's own risk. It is up to you whether you prefer to listen to a stupid doctor who is still licensed to practice, or to a pair of sensible ones who aren't! But we have more confidence in Mother Nature than in Medicine by Committee and by Numbers, and its consequent rigid medical practice. If we are right about the central role of Vitamin D in the normal immune response, then surely a more timely recognition of and response to the global epidemic of D-deficiency would have saved many lives and much distress from Covid-19.

We must remain concerned about the origins of the Covid-19 pandemic, It is not clear but it appears to have come from an animal reservoir, most likely bats, possibly pangolins. [Ref 35] In the prevention or control of an inevitable future pandemic, we maintain our proposition of improving human immune defence mechanisms by building up blood levels of Vitamin D with a target level of 40ng/ml (100nmol/L). We support controls over the use of wild animals as human food, but we would stop short of extermination of bats and pangolins.

Should Vitamin D also be given in severe cases?

When talking about Vitamin D for severely ill and recovering patients we are on more unsettled ground;

Vitamin D might then be unfairly blamed for death or any residual brain damage. We are all biochemically different, and there are many variants of the VDR that may make particular patients and particular tissues uniquely vulnerable to the combination of D-deficiency and coronavirus. On the other hand, maybe even Boris Johnson, who has said he was brought back from near death, owes his life to a sensible doctor who said, 'D is a Vitamin, it can't do you any harm, so let's just give it'! Much boils down to individual clinical judgement.

Remember *encephalitis lethargica*

It is worth recalling that there was a global epidemic that started during the first World War and continued episodically till 1926, of a serious generalised brain disease called *encephalitis lethargica*. [Ref 36] This reached a peak at the time of the 1918/19 influenza pandemic, to which it might have been connected but this is far from clear. It was associated in its late stages with a particularly severe form of Parkinsonism. The basal ganglia, which are concerned with movement, include the *substantia nigra*, which possesses the enzyme 1-alpha hydroxylase, and VDRs. (Refs 37, 38]. We mention this because in many severe cases of Covid-19 there are curious unexplained neurological symptoms. Jennifer Frontera, a New York hospital neurologist found that some patients started having unusual movements, some seizures and others strokes. Some neurological symptoms appear to be mild, such as the loss of smell and taste, but a few patients have developed encephalitis (Ref 39, 40]. It remains to be seen whether such features improve, stay static, or deteriorate if and when Vitamin D is given late; and whether as with *encephalitis lethargica* there might be a risk of late Parkinsonism or other serious brain sequelae.

Preparing better next time

Was the past three months really the best our Government and its appointed experts could do to face an entirely predictable global pandemic disaster? Such pessimism will become all the greater if, as we fear happened following the Foot and Mouth Disease epidemic of 20 years ago, not only are no lessons learnt, but the same advisers are retained to use modelling based on weak maths, a total ignorance of biology, and spin. But alas we fear that basic ignorance of science, coupled with undeclared conflicts of interest, may continue unchecked.

In the UK the situation is compounded by a high degree of British arrogance mixed with ignorance. All that matters is consensus, and the over-riding need to be right all the time. Within decision-making the current trick is to appoint large Committees that inevitably dilute the opinions of those who are intelligent, scientifically literate, and able to articulate the case for reason and common sense. There is little point in directing firepower at politicians for not having any scientific nouse, because we always knew that. But doctors and scientists should surely have had a better training and education? Over the past 30 years, has regimentation of medical education so reduced the freedom for the individual doctors to think for themselves? At the same time the medical-scientific input to public health bodies has diminished.

It seems that in debate, everything everywhere now hinges round the majority vote, however slender, as was seen with Brexit, with its ratio of 51.9 to 48.1%, and where blatant lies were permitted. We know that for Vitamin D, safe supplements are essential this far North for more than half the year; yet a Selected Committee consisting mainly of nutritionists, based on arguments that ignore the most fundamental roles of Vitamin D, has its decisions set in tablets of stone. And simplistic strategies are used by people with vested interests who are unwilling or unable to stand back and admit the obvious. Does anyone have the right to ignore billions of years of evolution for short-term profit?

An obvious major paradox

One of the most puzzling paradoxes in the Great Coronavirus D-bacle is the willingness of Governments worldwide to close their countries down, with devastating consequences for the World Economy, massive unemployment, and ruin for the aircraft industry.

Regardless, we fail to understand why there seems to be so little concern. Is it just a single lack of intelligence, or is there something more afoot? Time will tell whether, as believed by some on the basis of an apparent insertion into the coronavirus genome of 12 bases [Ref 41] there has indeed been an element of human genetic tampering. But we need to end this book on a more positive note.

Planning for the next Pandemic

It is to be hoped that the pandemic of Covid-19 will be used as a learning exercise, and there is much to be learned. We are not clear whether UK Government sponsored clinical research is taking place, but there is much concerning virus genome sequencing and vaccine development. Covid-19 is not the first pandemic, nor

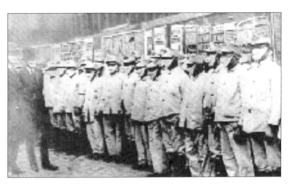

Spanish flu pandemic 1919

will it be the last. It is essential to prepare for the next epidemic in a more practical way than for the present one. What we would like to see is a concentration not on the virus itself, as it has not yet escaped from its animal reservoir, and it is completely unknown to us. To be told that 'Britain was blinded by the wrong virus' (*Guardian* May 22) [Ref 42] is rather like railways coming to a halt because of the 'wrong type of leaves on the tracks'. The value of the preparation for the pandemic ('the best in the world after the USA') should have been of equal benefit whether the virus turned out to be an influenza virus or a coronavirus.

We cannot pick and choose the virus of the next epidemic, but better preparation is essential, and Britain should surely lead the way. Planning should concentrate on protection of the next generation against the next virus, whatever it might be. Defence of the public should be independent of the virus, and should maximize immunity of everyone against any virus.

This protection should build on what natural selection and evolution have provided. This is Vitamin D, which appeared 1.5 billion years ago, and its immune modulating

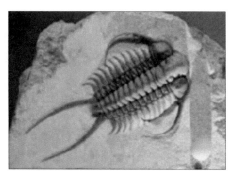

The Cambrian explosion of life 500M years ago:
Was it triggered by the evolution of the VDR that is
activated by Vitamin D?

function that developed 500 million years ago. We have explained how biomedical science during recent decades has given us great understanding of the ability of Vitamin D, together with cellular VDR, to escalate the defensive immune response when a serious infection occurs. So the plan should involve testing the Vitamin D status of the population and giving supplements to those deficient, which over winter means everyone. With a radiation exposure we would give iodine tablets. With a biological exposure we should give Vitamin D. New vaccines, if needed at all, should follow that.

We agree that a basic blood level of Vitamin D, as acknowledged by the government advice from SACN is needed; it is just that the current one is much too low to escalate defensive immunity in response to infection. Future pandemics cannot be predicted, so it is necessary for the population to be prepared now. Consideration is needed for forming a Scientific Committee for Immune Defence (SACID). We have explained that a blood level of 40ng/ml (100nmol/L) should be the target, but we anticipate that this level will at present be found only rarely. An annual blood test should be considered to make certain that the target blood level has been achieved. The Vitamin D supplement could be given conveniently in a number of ways: a daily dose of 4,000 units; a weekly dose of 20,000 units; or a monthly dose of 100,000 units. Whether funded by the NHS, or from personal income for those who can afford it, this is inexpensive.

Finally, there should be consideration of altering the UK sun-avoidance policy. This is defined by SACN [Ref 34], which sees vitamin D in terms of nutrition rather than as a pre-hormone produced in the skin. People should be encouraged to spend time in the sun without sunscreens, but without sunburn. Time control should be emphasised rather than sunscreen being applied before going outdoors, but with clothes or sunscreen being applied after a certain time. This will depend the time of the year, the time of the day, and the geographical location. There will be other proposals to reduce the impact of the next pandemic, but if we have learned one thing from Covid-19, it is that the preparation for it and the response to it have been woefully inadequate. Ignoring the immuno-protective role of The Sunshine Vitamin has been a serious, senseless, selfish and for many a fatal error.

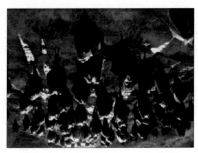

Bats

References

Ref 1

Anderson DC. *Where Angels Fear to Tread – my life in Medicine and minding other people's business.* Authorhouse 2018.

Ref 2

Anderson DC. *Hongshan Jade Treasures: The Art, Iconography and Authentication of Carvings from China's finest Neolithic Culture.* Editrice Tau, 2012.

Ref 3

Anderson DC, Scott NP. *Three False Convictions, Many Lessons: The Psychopathology of Unjust Prosecutions.* Waterside Press 2016.

Ref 4

Grimes DS. *Vitamin D and Cholesterol: the importance of the sun.* YPD-BOOKS, 2009.

Ref 5

DG Blog
http://www.drdavidgrimes.com/2020/05/covid-19-vitamin-d-and-uk-government.html

Ref 6

Hanel A, Carlberg C. *Vitamin D and evolution: pharmacologic implications*. Biochemical Pharmacology 2020; 173: https://doi.org/10.1016/j.bcp.2019.07.024

Ref 7

Ferguson, Margaret. *A study of social and economic factors in the causation of rickets, with introductory historical survey by Leonard Findlay*. London 1918. Medical Research Council Special Report Series, Number 20.

Ref 8

Hutchison HS, Shah SJ. *The aetiology of rickets, early and late*. Quarterly Journal of Medicine 1922. 15: 167–194

Ref 9

Hobday R. *Healing Sun: Sunshine and Health in the 21st Century*. Inner Traditions/Bear, 2000.

Ref 10

Green M. *Cod liver oil and tuberculosis*. Br Med J 2011; 343: d7505

Ref 11

Chun RF, Liu PT, Modlin RL, Adams JS, Hewison M. *Impact of vitamin D on immune function: lessons learned from genome-wide analysis*. Front Physiol 2014; 5: 151.   10.3389/fphys.2014.00151

Ref 12

McGrath MS, Kodelja V. *Balanced macrophage activation hypothesis: a biological model for development of drugs targeted at macrophage functional states.* Pathobiology 1999; 67: 277–81

Ref 13

Zhan Y, Leung DYM, Richers BN et al. *Vitamin D Inhibits Monocyte/macrophage Pro-inflammatory Cytokine Production by Targeting Mitogen-Activated Protein Kinase Phosphatase 1.* J Immunol. 2012 Mar 1; 188: 2127–2135.

Ref 14

The Vitamin D Levels of the Hadzabe and the Maasai: An Important Study That Flew Under the Radar. Darwinian Medicine maasaihttp://darwinian-medicine.com/the-vitamin-d-levels-of-the-hadzabe-and-the-maasai-an-important-study-that-flew-under-the-radar/

Ref 15

Raharusuna P, Priambada S, Budiarti C, Agung E, Budi C. *Patterns of COVID-19 Mortality and Vitamin D: An Indonesian Study.* https://papers.ssrn.com/sol3/papers.cfm?abstract_id=3585561 Disclaimer: This is a preliminary study for early dissemination of results. Data are subject to changes.

Ref 16

Alipio M. *Vitamin D Supplementation Could Possibly Improve Clinical Outcomes of Patients Infected with Coronavirus-2019 (COVID-19).*
https://papers.ssrn.com/sol3/papers.cfm?abstract_id=3571484

Ref 17

Glicio EJ. *Vitamin D Level of Mild and Severe Elderly Cases of COVID-19: A Preliminary Report.* (This is preliminary report)
https://papers.ssrn.com/sol3/papers.cfm?abstract_id=3593258#.XrE0oF1wSjU.twitter

Ref 18

Deaths involving COVID-19, England and Wales: deaths occurring in April 2020. Released May 15th 2020
https://www.ons.gov.uk/peoplepopulationandcommunity/birthsdeathsandmarriages/deaths/bulletins/deathsinvolvingcovid19englandandwales/deathsoccurringinapril2020

Ref 19

mats.humble@oru.se; susanne.bejerot@oru.se

Ref 20

Thomas Kuhn. *The structure of Scientific Revolutions.* Chicago and London. Fourth Edition, page 93.

Ref 21

Death of Dr El Tayar
https://www.bbc.co.uk/news/uk-england-london-52064450

Ref 22

https://www.lancashiretelegraph.co.uk/news/18388799.e-lancs-doctor-high-rate-black-ethnic-minority-coronavirus-deaths-national-crisis/

Ref 23

https://www.ons.gov.uk/peoplepopulationandcommunity/birthsdeathsandmarriages/deaths/bulletins/deathsinvolvingcovid19bylocalareasanddeprivation/deathsoccurringbetween1marchand17april

Ref 24

https://www.england.nhs.uk/wp-content/uploads/2020/05/valabhji-COVID-19-and-Diabetes-Paper-1.pdf

Ref 25

https://diabetes.diabetesjournals.org/content/57/10/2565

Ref 26

Arnljots R, Thorn J, Elm M, Moore M, Sundvall P. Vitamin D deficiency was common among nursing home residents and associated with dementia: a cross sectional study of 545 Swedish nursing home residents. BMC Geriatrics 2017; 17: 299.
https://bmcgeriatr.biomedcentral.com

Ref 27

Schwalfenberg G. *Vitamin D supplementation in a nursing home population*. Molecular Nutrition & Food Research 54: 8.
https://onlinelibrary.wiley.com/doi/abs/10.1002/mnfr.200900601

Ref 28

The National Heart, Lung, and Blood Institute PETAL Clinical Trials Network Early High-Dose Vitamin D_3 for Critically ill, Vitamin D-Deficient Patients
N Engl J Med 2019;381:2529-40.

Ref 29

Lucas RM, McMichael AJ
Association or Causation: evaluating links between "environment and disease"
Public Health Classics
Bulletin of the World Health Organization October 2005, 83 (10)
https://www.who.int/bulletin/volumes/83/10/792.pdf

Ref 30

Doll R, Hill AB. *Mortality in Relation to Smoking: Ten Years' Observations of British Doctors*. Br Med J 1964; 1 (5395): 1399–1410.

Ref 31

https://www.publichealth.hscni.net/news/pha-recommends-daily-vitamin-d-supplement-during-lockdown

Ref 32

Beeley V.
https://off-guardian.org/2020/05/10/covid19-the-big-pharma-players-behind-uk-government-lockdown/

Ref 33

https://www.narcolepsy.org.uk/resources/pandemrix-narcolepsy

Ref 34

Vitamin D and Health. 2016. Scientific Advisory Committee on Nutrition UK Government.
https://assets.publishing.service.gov.uk/government/uploads/system/uploads/attachment_data/file/537616/SACN_Vitamin_D_and_Health_report.pdf

Ref 35

Andersen KG, Rambaut A, Lipkin WI, Holmes EC, Garry RF. *The proximal origin of SARS-CoV-2.* Nature Medicine 2020; 26: 450–452.

Ref 36

Encephalitis lethargica.
https://academic.oup.com/brain/article/140/8/2246/3970828

Ref 37

Eyles DW, Smith S, Kinobe R, Hewisn M, McGrath JJ. *Distribution of the Vitamin D receptor and 1α-hydroxylase in human brain.* Journal of Chemical Neuroanatomy 2005; 29: 21–30. 10.1016/j.jchemneu.2004.08.006

Ref 38

Cui X, Pelekanos M, Liu P–Y, Burne THJ, McGrath JJ, Eyles DW. *The Vitamin D Receptor in Dopamine Neurons; Its Presence in Human Substantia Nigra and Its Ontogenesis in Rat Midbrain.* J Neuroscience 2013. 10.1016/j.neuroscience.2013.01.035

Ref 39

Hamzelou J. Virus on the brain. New Scientist 2020, May 30. Pages 35–38.
https://www.newscientist.com/article/mg24632842-800-coronavirus-seems-to-reach-the-brain-what-could-this-mean-for-us/#ixzz6Npxs3dOb

Ref 40

Hughes D. The patients who just can't shake off Covid-19.
https://www.bbc.com/news/health-52548843

Ref 41

Genome of Covid-19
https://www.sciencedirect.com/science/article/pii/S1684118220300827

Ref 42

https://www.theguardian.com/world/2020/may/21/did-the-uk-government-prepare-for-the-wrong-kind-of-pandemic

Appendix 1

The Sunshine Vitamin's Lament
by Dr David C Anderson

D-one, D-two, but where's D-three?
And what's this UV ABC?
The sun shines on the empty beach
The President just trumpets 'bleach'
While Covid kills for free

Test anywhere, you'll find D's lack,
Our priest in Italy is black:
If ignorance is bliss for some
For others it spells 'Kingdom Come'
The crown will call you back

We all need D, but where's the proof?
Deficiency might be a spoof
With every Bamey doctor's death
We shake our heads and save our breath
While testing hits the roof

Agog, we 'wait the next absurd
Pronouncement 'pon the waiting herd;
Advisers hold our life in balance
Chris Whitty and yer Patrick Vallance
Barge forth quite under turd

We'll stick to social distancing
And let the dead go disc-dancing
With kingdom Cummings up on high
Alert: since BJ failed to die
They'll do this Brexit thing

Committees do not like big numbers
I fear it shakes them from their slumbers:
One hundred thousand's lots of noughts
Four hundred daily's more their torts
So onward they just lumber

We feel the regulator's sighs
He really cares for our demise
Blue gloves and dirty masks of death
No PPEs? - just save your breath
Cock-handed Matt is wise!

Does no one see the irony
In thorny blobs of RNA!
They'll save the NHS indoors
Speak platitudes until it boors
To death, to get their way

What? Problem-solving with a vial
The blindest fool needs blinded trial!
I lie in bed and dream my dreams
But no one hears my silent screams;
Black death may last awhile

Appendix 2

I had a Dream
by David Grimes

Day 0 (May 2020)
The scene: *The Press Room, 10 Downing Street, London W1*

The reporters are waiting, now on-line.
Enter three men, and stand behind their lecterns.

Prime Minister, Boris Johnson

This morning we have, er, some very good news for you all. I will ask Chris Whitty to give more details.

Professor Chris Whitty, Chief Medical Officer

Thank you Prime Minister. The good news today is that we now have a new way to reduce dramatically serious illness and deaths from Covid-19. The way to do this is actually simple and it is available immediately. We have heard a great deal about the development of vaccines to provide immunity, but it is unlikely that they will be available and tested for safety until the end of the year. In the meantime we have a great opportunity. It is vitamin D. It will boost our immunity and reduce deaths at a stroke (© Edward Heath).

Prime Minister

So there we are. I told you that we had really good news today, great news. I will turn to Patrick to explain further.

Sir Patrick Vallance, Chief Scientist

Thank you Prime Minister. Vitamin D is not new. In fact it first appeared on the evolutionary scale 1.2 billion years ago, but its importance in immunity has been a feature of only the past 500 million years. The next bit is slightly technical. Vitamin D is created by the action of the sun on 7-dehydro-cholesterol that is manufactured in our skin. It becomes activated in the liver and kidneys and, combining with vitamin D receptors (VDRs) on the cell surface, it activates several genes. These include genes that enable the proliferation in response to infection of the defensive immunity cells, such as T-lymphocytes and macrophages.

Prime Minister

I think I can just about understand that. Would you like to add anything Chris?

Chris Whitty

It was realised early in the 20th century that vitamin D was important for immunity. At that time rickets was common in our industrial cities and this was shown to be due to shortage of vitamin D, the result of air pollution preventing the penetration of full intensity sunlight to ground level. It was noted that rickets and tuberculosis frequently co-existed within families. It is now clear from the experience of the AIDS epidemic in particular that tuberculosis becomes activated when immunity is suppressed.

Prime Minister

Do you mean that air pollution causes suppression of immunity?

Patrick Vallance

Yes, and in the pandemic of Covid-19 we have seen that it took hold in northern Italy, which has the greatest air pollution in Europe and where blood level of vitamin D are particularly low. It will also explain why the pandemic is causing more deaths in our inner cities than in rural areas

Prime Minister

There is more evidence concerning the value of vitamin D in Covid-19.

Patrick Vallance

Yes. It is possible to measure the amount of vitamin D in the body by a simple blood test that has been available in all NHS hospitals for several years, and it is available in many countries in the world. It is important for the blood level of vitamin D to be greater than 30ng/ml, or 75nmol/L. Less than 10 is regarded as serious deficiency. An imaginative study has been reported from the Philippines by Professor Mark Alipiorrt, who unfortunately has been very ill with pneumonia, but I am told that he is now recovering. Vitamin D testing was undertaken in 212 patients with proven Covid-19 in three hospitals in south-east Asia.

Prime Minister

Chris, can you tell us the results?

Chris Whitty

The results are dramatic. Of the 55 patients with ideal blood levels of vitamin D, 47 had just mild disease. In 4 the disease was moderate, in 2 severe and in 2 critical. But on the other hand, in the 157 patients with low blood levels of vitamin D, only 2 had mild disease, and in the other 155 patients the disease was moderate, severe or critical.

Prime Minister

Gosh! So there was a clear benefit from having a good blood level of vitamin D. I think there has been another study. Patrick.

Patrick Vallance

Yes Prime Minister. This was in Indonesia. As the pandemic started in the far East, there have been more opportunities for research. 780 patients with Covid-19 were tested for blood levels of vitamin D, and they were followed up to observe clinical outcome. Chris.

Chris Whitty

Almost half of the patients had low levels of vitamin D, and almost half of the patients died. Of the 380 with good levels of vitamin D, that is above 30, only 16 died. Of the 400 with low levels of vitamin D, almost all died.

Prime Minister

This is really amazing. Are there any other studies?

Chris Whitty

Yes. I have just received this morning a report from an imaginative Dr Gerry Schwalfenberg in Edmonton, Alberta, in Canada. He realised a little while ago that low blood vitamin D level is a bad thing and especially common in elderly people living in care homes. He looks after residents in a nursing home and so he gave them all vitamin D 2,000units each day by mouth and later he tested the blood levels. in 94% of the residents, the levels were above 32ng/ml (80nmol/L). Those whose blood levels remained low were given a higher dose of vitamin D.

Prime Minister

Has that been of benefit to them?

Chris Whitty

Yes it has. Not a single resident of this nursing home has been ill with Covid-19, whereas there have been many cases in all the other neighbouring nursing homes

Prime Minister

That is even more really good news. Are there any more examples, Chris?

Chris Whitty

Yes. With exception of San Marino, Belgium has in Europe the highest number of Cid-19 deaths relative to population size. We have just the morning read a report from Belgium that vitamin D levels are much lower in the patients who died from Covid-19.

Prime Minister

So we have a great opportunity to protect the wonderful and proud people of our great country, and defeat the most dangerous enemy that we have faced since the second world war. Patrick, what is the next step?

Patrick Vallance

We have these clinical studies and we have the basic science of the vital role of vitamin D in the process of immunity. We need to protect people by issuing them with vitamin D. There are two dosage regimes. The first is to use capsules or tablets of vitamin D. A dose of 2,000 units a day is usually adequate, but at this time of national emergency I would recommend 4,000 units a day. An alternative is to give a single dose of 100,000 units, in an oil which can be given by injection or by mouth. Its effect will last for about two months.

Prime Minister

Will this be expensive? Do we need to ask the permission of the Chancellor of the Exchequer?

Patrick Vallance

It is cheap. The single dose will cost about £1, and the 4,000 unit capsules will cost about £10 for a year's supply. We obviously must multiply these numbers by the number of the UK population.

Prime Minister

That is even more good news. I am sure that our Chancellor of the Exchequer Rashi Sunak will be very pleased. Chris, do you have any comments?

Chris Whitty

It will take a little time for the public health departments in the UK to organise the distribution of vitamin D.

Prime Minister

But surely this is very urgent. People are still dying from Covid-19, about 500 each day.

Chris Whitty

Yes, and we need to prioritise distribution to those most at risk. This will obviously be health service workers, and then care workers, and then the residents of care homes.

Prime Minister

I think that I might have heard a suggestion that people of black African and Asian ethnicity might be at risk from Covid-19. Patrick, do you know if this might be true?

Patrick Vallance

I might have also have heard the suggestion that people of black African and Asian ethnicity might be at special risk. There is a view that they must all be rehoused as a matter of urgency. I am also given to understand, but I have not seen any official figures, that 25 of the 26 UK doctors who have died from Covid-19 were of black African and

Asian ethnicity. It has been known for a long time that such people are almost all deficient in vitamin D as the result of dark skin and sun-avoiding behaviour.

Prime Minister

And so must they also have a priority for receiving vitamin D?

Sir Patrick Vallance

Yes, Prime Minister. But the more people who have priority, the more difficult the task of distribution.

Prime Minister

But if the vitamin is so cheap people might want to buy their own supplies.

Chris Whitty

Yes Prime Minister, that is what I have done.

Sir Patrick Vallance

And so have I.

Prime Minister

I think I was given an injection of vitamin D when I was in hospital

Chris Whitty

That is probably why you recovered so well and so quickly when you were so close to death.

Prime Minister

Yes, and once again I would like to thank all the brave staff for the wonderful treatment and care that I was given. So, the vitamin D story seems to be straightforward.. Are there any dissenting voices?

Patrick Vallance

There are a few. Notably the Oxford group, who are busy developing and testing a vaccine. They feel that vitamin D is an untested diversion from what they are doing.

Chris Whitty

And there are many who feel that social justice for the ethnic and socio-economically disadvantaged should have priority over vitamin D supplements.

Prime Minister

That is tricky. So I think we must go ahead with vitamin D immediately. Today at the latest. Are there any questions? Laura.

Laura Keuensberg (BBC)

Thank you all for this welcome news.

Could I please ask where vitamin D supplements come from and is there an adequate supply?

Prime Minister

Patrick, this is one for you.

Patrick Vallance

Thank you Laura. Most of the vitamin D supplements come from sheep's wool, and some from fish oil. The oil from sheep's wool must be processed to isolate 7-dehydro-cholesterol, and then this must be irradiated with UV light to convert it into vitamin D. A possible problem is that the great majority of this production takes place in China. I believe the world annual production is about 7 million tonnes. Most of it goes into animal feed, very important now that so many animals are kept indoors. The UK might require about 1 million tonnes.

Prime Minister

Thank you Laura. Beth, you have a question.

Beth Rigby (Sky News)

You have mentioned the Oxford group who are inventing a vaccine at this moment. I am told that they demand a randomised control trial to see if there is any truth in the idea that vitamin D might be helpful in Covid-19. Is a trial under way in the UK?

Prime Minister

Patrick should be able to answer this one.

Patrick Vallance

I do not have a full picture of any research that is going on at present. Perhaps Chris would know more.

Chris Whitty

I do not know of any, but any research that individual hospitals do is up to themselves. The information about vitamin D that I have is that common sense tells us how good it is, and that is why I take it. If we have a controlled trial, half the subjects will take vitamin D and half will take a placebo, a dummy tablet. I would not be happy for me or any of my family or friends (with an occasional exception) to take the placebo as it might put me or others at a high risk of death. Unless we keep the subjects in the dark (perhaps literally) I do not see a controlled trial taking place. In other words at this stage, to conduct a placebo controlled trial of vitamin D with informed consent would not be ethical. The weight of evidence for vitamin D to be helpful in preventing serious illness and death from Covid-19 is well beyond reasonable doubt, to use a legal expression. We know that vitamin D is safe, but we do not yet have this information about the Oxford Vaccine.

Prime Minister

Thanks you Chris. That is very clear.Heather, you have a question.

Heather Stewart (Guardian)

We hear great deal about testing. How many people in the UK have had their blood vitamin D levels tested?

Prime Minister

Chris, can you answer this?

Chris Whitty

The short answer is that I have no idea. Hospitals do not inform the centre about the blood tests that they undertake.

Prime Minister

Thank you Heather. I think you have another question

Heather Stewart

Yes Prime Minister. Thank you. At the Guardian I am told that during the past month we have had a lot of letters about the value of vitamin D in the pandemic, mainly written by doctors. We published just one letter but we thought that the others must be from food-fad enthusiasts. Do you mean to say that they were all right in what they had written to us?

Prime Minister

Patrick, you might answer this.

Patrick Vallance

Well, Heather, it looks as though they were right.

Prime Minister

Tim, you have question.

Tim Shipman (Times & Sunday Times)

It sound as though there might be widespread knowledge of the value of vitamin D in immunity and defence against infection. We have just heard about it for the first time this morning, and so may I ask when you first heard about it?

Prime Minister

Speaking for myself, it was just after breakfast this morning. What about you Patrick?

Patrick Vallance

I heard about it yesterday evening. I was alerted by a member of staff who had just seen some interesting Blog posts and Emails.

Prime Minister

And you Chris ? When did you first hear about it?

Chris Whitty

When Patrick phoned me yesterday evening.

Tim Shipman

Why did you as Chief Medical Officer not know about the value of vitamin D in defensive immunity?

Chris Whitty

Well, I can't be expected to know everything. I thought vitamin D was all about bones and children with rickets. The importance for immunity is new to me.

Prime Minister

Let's move on. Bob, you have a question.

Robert Peston (ITV News)

Prime Minister, what can people do if supplies of vitamin D are not sufficient for our needs?

Prime Minister

That is difficult one Bob. Over to you Patrick.

Patrick Vallance

We can eat oily fish, such as mackerel in particular. Do you remember the days when as children we were given disgusting Cod Liver Oil? It turns out that our mothers were right. We can also obtain vitamin D from the sun, and in fact we obtain most of our vitamin D from the sun. We need to expose our skin, not quite all of it, to the sun, at this time of the year in the UK up to an hour between 10:00am and 4:00pm. We can do this in our gardens, in the parks, and on the beach, or anywhere that is isn't too cold, and of course when it is not raining.

Prime Minister

That might be bit tricky with social distancing, but we must act very quickly. I suppose we might do what I believe is happening in supermarkets and other places. People would apply for a ticket to lie semi-naked in a park (not in a supermarket) or on a beach so that there are not too many people in one place at one time. We would need to have police on patrol. We should be able to create a web-site for it this evening and set this up by tomorrow morning. Are there any more questions?

Goes on for another half hour with the usual questions and usual evasive answers.

Day 1

Daily Covid-19 briefing becomes chaotic as Matt Hancock (Secretary of State for Health), Angel McLean (Deputy Chief Scientific Advisor), and Jenny Harries (Deputy Chief Medical Officer) are inundated with questions about vitamin D that they are unable to answer.

The briefing is brought to a rapid close.

Newspaper headlines:

All hospital patients with Covid-19 given Vitamin D

Crowds outside pharmacies

Vitamin D is in short supply

Demand for permits is overwhelming

Web-site for permits to sunbathe in public places crashes.

Public parks crowded with semi-naked people

Queues of cars at approaches to beaches

Asian groups complain that sunbathing advice is against their religious practices

Day 2

Newspaper headlines:

Government suspends daily Covid-19 announcements

Vitamin D supplies to the public are exhausted

Black market develops for vitamin D

People fighting for entry into parks

Sunbathers refuse to leave after one hour

Police cannot control crowds

Day 3

Newspaper headlines:

Public Health agencies are struggling to prioritise the
vitamin D supplies that they have been able to obtain.
China refuses to release more vitamin D

It is not yet warm enough to shear sheep

Fish shops noting a big demand for mackerel

Day 4

Newspaper headlines:

Vitamin D : Civil disobedience.
Family doctors are struggling with demand for
vitamin D blood tests
Crowds outside hospitals demanding vitamin D
Heavy rain diminishes crowds in parks

Day 5

Newspaper headlines:

Why was vitamin D not stockpiled?
If vitamin D has been known for a long time to help
immunity,
why was it not recommended two months ago?
Large protests in Trafalgar Square
Chief Medical Officer and Chief Scientist resign
Calls on Prime Minister to resign

Day 6

Newspaper headlines:

Sudden end of deaths from Covid-19
Lockdown ended to enable to people go outside to work or to sunbathe

Day 7

Newspaper headlines:

In anticipation of future epidemics, Government sets up Scientific Advisory Committee for Immune Defence

And then I woke up, listened to the radio news and I realised that it had all been a dream, but a pleasant dream. It would have been nice to remain asleep but now I was awake I had to continue with the daily nightmare of Covid-19 with no action taken to stop deaths. How many more will die today?

Appendix 3

Doctors who died from Covid-19

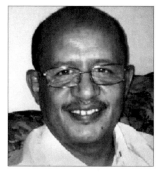

*Dr Adil El Tatar – Age 63
Died March 25th*

*Organ transplant surgeon
who was volunteering
to work in A&E in the
Midlands*

Dr Adil El Tatar

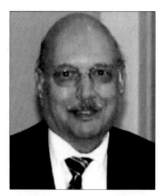

*Dr Habib Zaidi – Age 76
Died March 25th*

*General Practitioner
working in the Eastwood
Group Practice, Essex*

Dr Habib Zaidi

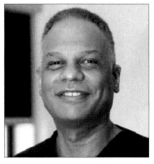

Dr Amged El-Hawrani

Dr Amged El-Hawrani
– Age 55
Died March 28th

ENT Consultant
Queen's Hospital,
Burton-on-Trent

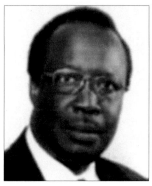

Dr Eric Labeja-Acellan

Dr Eric Labeja-Acellan
– Age 69
Died March 31st

Consultant,
University Hospital,
Lewisham, London

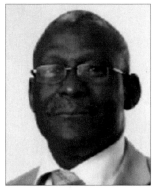

Dr Alfa Saadu

Dr Alfa Saadu – Age 68
Died March 31st

Former Consultant and
Medical Director,
Essex and Ealing

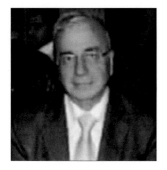

Dr Sami Shousha

*Dr Sami Shousha – Age 79
Died April 2ⁿᵈ*

*Consultant Histopathologist,
Charing Cross Hospital,
London*

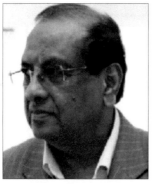

Dr Anton Sebastianpillai

*Dr Anton Sebastianpillai
– Age 70s
Died April 4ᵗʰ*

*Consultant Geriatrician,
Kingston Hospital, London*

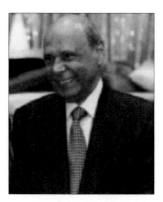

Dr Syed Zishan Haider

*Dr Syed Zishan Haider
– Age 79
Died April 4ᵗʰ*

*General Practioner,
Valence Medical Centre,
Dagenham*

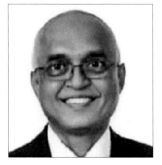

Dr Jitendra Rathod – Age 62
Died April 6th

Consultant Heart Surgeon,
Cardiff

Dr Jitendra Rathod

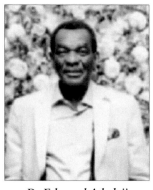

Dr Edmond Adedeji – Age 62
Died April 8th

Locum Registrar,
A&E Department
Great Western Hospital

Dr Edmond Adedeji

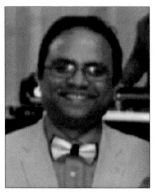

Dr Abdul Mabud Chowdhury
– Age 53
Died April 8th

Consultant Urologist,
Homerton Hospital, London

Dr Abdul Mabud
Chowdhury

131

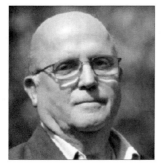

Dr Fayez Ayache

Dr Fayez Ayache – Age 76
Died April 8ᵗʰ

General Practitioner in
Suffolk and Essex

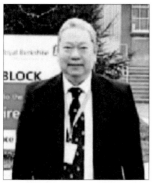

Dr Peter Tun

Dr Peter Tun – Age 62
Died April 13ᵗʰ

Associate Specialist in
Neuro-rehabilitation,
Royal Berkshire Hospital,
Reading

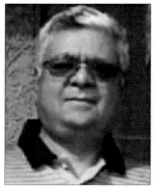

Dr Rajesh Kalraiya

Dr Rajesh Kalraiya – Age 70
Died April 15ᵗʰ

Consultant Paediatrician,
Noth-East London

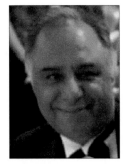

Dr Krishnan Arora – Age 57
Died April 15th

General Practitioner,
Violet Lane Medical Practice,
Croydon

Dr Krishnan Arora

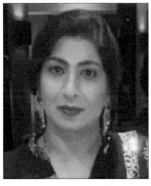

Dr Mamoona Rana – Age 48
Died April 16th

Trainee in Psychiatry,
North East London

Dr Mamoona Rana

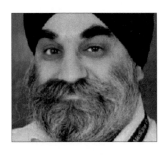

Dr Manjeet Singh Riya
– Age 52
Died April 20th

Consultant in
Emergency Medicine,
Royal Derby Hospital

Dr Manjeet Singh Riya

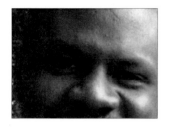

Dr Muhaned Nowa Eltayib

Dr Muhaned Nowa Eltayib
Died April 20th

Registrar, Royal Victoria
Hospital, Belfast

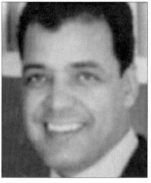

Dr Sadeq Elhowsh

Dr Sadeq Elhowsh – Age 58
Died April 20th

Consultant Orthopaedic
Surgeon,
St Helen's & Knowsely
Hospitals

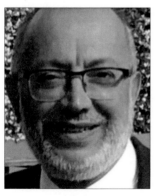

Dr Yusuf Patel

Dr Yusuf Patel
Died April 22nd

General Practitioner,
Forest Gate, London

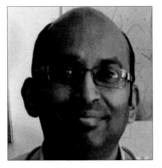

Dr Vishna Rasiah

Dr Vishna Rasiah

*Consultant Neonatal
Paediatrician,
Midlands*

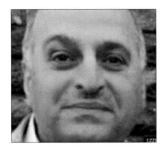

Dr Saad Al-Dubbaisi

*Dr Saad Al-Dubbaisi
– Age 59
Died May 2nd*

*General Practitioner,
Garden City Medical Centre,
Ramsbottom*

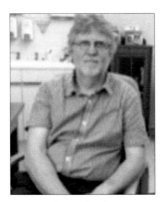

Dr Craig Wakeham

Dr Craig Wakeham

*General Practitioner, Carne
Abbas Surgery, Dorset*

*The only non-BAME doctor
to have died from Covid-19*